Care *of* Children Exposed *to the* Traumatic Effects *of* Disaster

T0176408

Care *of* Children Exposed *to the* Traumatic Effects *of* Disaster

by

Jon A. Shaw, M.D., M.S.

Zelde Espinel, M.D., M.A., M.P.H.

James M. Shultz, M.S., Ph.D.

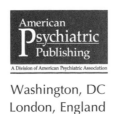

American Psychiatric Publishing
A Division of American Psychiatric Association

Washington, DC
London, England

If you would like to buy between 25 and 99 copies of this or any other American Psychiatric Publishing title, you are eligible for a 20% discount; please contact Customer Service at appi@psych.org or 800-368-5777. If you wish to buy 100 or more copies of the same title, please e-mail us at bulksales@psych.org for a price quote.

Copyright © 2012 American Psychiatric Association

ALL RIGHTS RESERVED

Manufactured in the United States of America on acid-free paper

15   14   13   12   11   5   4   3   2   1

First Edition

Typeset in Adobe's Book Antiqua and Optima.

American Psychiatric Publishing
1000 Wilson Boulevard
Arlington, VA 22209–3901
www.appi.org

Library of Congress Cataloging-in-Publication Data
Shaw, Jon A.
  Care of children exposed to the traumatic effects of disaster / by Jon A. Shaw, Zelde Espinel, James M. Shultz. — 1st ed.
    p. ; cm.
  Includes bibliographical references and index.
  ISBN 978-1-58562-426-3 (pbk. : alk. paper)
  I. Espinel, Zelde, 1966– II. Shultz, James M., 1950– III. American Psychiatric Publishing. IV. Title.
  [DNLM: 1. Child Psychology. 2. Stress, Psychological—psychology.
3. Child Welfare. 4. Disasters. 5. Emergencies—psychology. WS 350]
  618.92′89–dc23

                                                        2011043244

British Library Cataloguing in Publication Data
A CIP record is available from the British Library.

Contents

About the Authors

Jon A. Shaw, M.D., M.S., is Professor of Psychiatry and Behavioral Sciences, Chief of Child and Adolescent Psychiatry and Behavioral Sciences, and Professor of Clinical Pediatrics in the Department of Psychiatry and Behavioral Sciences at the Miller School of Medicine of the University of Miami in Miami, Florida.

Zelde Espinel, M.D., M.A., M.P.H., is Co-Director of the Center for Disaster and Extreme Event Preparedness (DEEP Center) in the Department of Epidemiology and Public Health at the Miller School of Medicine of the University of Miami in Miami, Florida.

James M. Shultz, M.S., Ph.D., is Director of the Center for Disaster and Extreme Event Preparedness (DEEP Center) in the Department of Epidemiology and Public Health at the Miller School of Medicine of the University of Miami in Miami, Florida.

The authors of this book indicated that they have no competing interests or affiliations to declare.

Preface

One can empathize with the poet William Wordsworth who wrote, "The world is too much with us." People are bombarded almost on a daily basis with news of natural disasters, nuclear accidents, civil strife, ongoing threats of war, and conflicts between nations. Tragically, children and their families are often the victims. This book is an effort to bring together our understanding of the effects of disaster on children and their families and the various means available for helping them in their hour of need. Although children are generally exposed to the same spectrum of hazards as adults, they are still maturing physically, emotionally, cognitively, and socially. Thus, the impact of perceived threat or physical harm must be understood in terms of the child's developmental level and also within the family and social context in which the child lives.

A recent survey of a representative sample of 2,030 children, ages 2–17 years, in the United States indicates that the lifetime exposure to disaster is 13.9% and that 4.1% of the children had experienced a disaster in the preceding year (Becker-Blease et al. 2010). Copeland et al. (2007) estimated that between 25% and 67% of children will be exposed to a significant traumatic event before reaching adulthood.

The National Commission on Children and Disasters (2010) recognizes the unique vulnerability of children to disaster, noting their cognitive and emotional immaturity and their elevated risk for emotional and behavioral problems, including posttraumatic stress disorder (PTSD), depression, anxiety, bereavement, academic failure, delinquency, and substance abuse. The commission indicates that the psychological consequences and mental health effects of disasters are frequently not prioritized in disaster management. Mental health and psychosocial support is typically omitted or provided in a delayed and suboptimal manner during response and recovery efforts. The commission further notes that postdisaster, children and families have limited access to mental health and treatment services. Consequently, "communities depend on persons who are not mental health professionals but who routinely interact with children—such as teachers and school staff, first responders, health care professionals, child care and early education providers, child welfare and juvenile justice professionals, and members of the faith-based community — to provide basic support services and brief interventions" (p. 35). These individuals need to be provided the skills necessary to recognize children in distress, to actively support positive coping skills, to monitor children's well-being in the aftermath of disaster, and to identify those who need more intensive evaluation and intervention. Our manual provides a knowledge base that will be helpful for the broad spectrum of professional and volunteer disaster responders who care for children affected by disasters.

Disasters, whether natural or human generated, involve an encounter between forces of harm and a human population in harm's way (Shultz et al. 2007). One hears almost daily the horrific accounts of the effects of natural disasters and extreme events, including earthquakes, tsunamis, monsoonal rains, flooding, blizzards, tornadoes, hurricanes, and droughts. As if the acts of nature were not enough, one increasingly sees the derivative effects of human-generated violence. Wars, civil strife, ethnic conflict, and acts of terrorism encircle the globe. Acts of terrorism against the United States have occurred in recent history and will occur again.

Millions of children are growing up in families and communities torn apart by armed conflict. In 1997, UNICEF reported that in the preceding decade, 2 million children had been killed in wars, 5 million had been disabled, and 12 million had been left homeless. However, these data probably misrepresent the true consequences of war on children. For example, half of the approximately 5.4 million deaths in the war in the Democratic Republic of the Congo were thought to be children (UNICEF 2009).

The child's psychological reactions to disaster are shaped by the unique forces of harm inherent in each type of disaster, as well as the degree of life threat and physical injury. In this book, we define terms essential to understanding the psychological effects of being exposed to disaster, such as *stress, primary and secondary stressors, acute traumatic moment,* and *traumatic reminders.* We note that the child's psychological responses to disaster occur across a timeline. These responses resonate with the impact phase and the cascade of secondary adversities in the aftermath of disaster and the complex array of contextual factors operating at individual, family, community, and societal levels. As a general benchmark for the postimpact phase, the acute or immediate phase lasts approximately 3–6 months, the intermediate phase lasts 6–18 months, and the longer, sustained recovery period may extend 2–5 years.

The child's psychological reaction is determined by individual factors such as age, gender, race, educational level, medical and psychiatric history, trauma history, and the child's level of functioning before and during the disaster. Powerful predictors of the child's response to disaster are family variables such as family structure, cohesiveness, communication patterns, parental response to disaster, and the family's postdisaster level of functioning. Salient community and societal factors include culture, ethnicity, socioeconomic status, social support, and postdisaster community functioning.

When a community is impacted by disaster, some identifiable groups of children will require additional, customized, or specialized approaches to assure their protection and to facilitate their recovery from the extreme event (Flynn 2006). Children with special needs include children who are developmentally disabled, children who are medically or psychiatrically ill, children living in poverty, foster care children, and children who have suffered from repetitive exposure to interpersonal violence or maltreatment.

Survivors of disaster are frequently exposed not only to individuals with life-threatening injuries but also to scenes of cruel and violent death. Children may suffer not only from exposure to the loss of family members but also concomitantly from exposure to their traumatic deaths. These children are said to suffer from child traumatic grief. Psychological and physiological reactions to bereavement (the fact of loss through death) are processed differently by children than by adults because of the children's cognitive, emotional, and physical immaturity. We discuss various strategies for support and intervention for the bereaved child.

Timely assessment and intervention are essential to mitigate the child's risk for ongoing distress, impairment, and psychiatric illness following traumatic exposure to disaster. We discuss the various parameters for understanding the psychological responses to trauma and disaster, as well as the procedures for a careful ongoing clinical assessment of children's and families' psychological reactions. As research on traumatized children and their families has increased, so has the level of thoughtfulness regarding psychosocial interventions to facilitate recovery.

Psychological reactions to disaster evolve or dissipate across a timeline through the postdisaster and recovery phases. Increasingly, emphasis is given to evidence-informed interventions to reduce psychological morbidity in the aftermath of disaster. One of these interventions is Psychological First Aid (National Child Traumatic Stress Network and National Center for PTSD 2006), an early intervention that is implemented in the immediate aftermath of disaster and was designed to reduce the initial distress and to foster adaptive coping for survivors of all ages. More recently, Skills for Psychological Recovery (Berkowitz et al. 2010) has been proposed as an evidence-informed intervention to be implemented in the intermediate phase following the application of Psychological First Aid to facilitate positive coping with postdisaster stressors and adversities. Other available interventions during the intermediate phase include psychoeducation, crisis intervention, cognitive-behavioral therapy, bereavement counseling, social supports, and psychopharmacology when indicated. Effective therapeutic intervention restores function and enhances recovery; creates a safe and secure environment; reduces uncertainty, fear, and anxiety; and mobilizes family and social supports.

Working with children exposed to traumatic events is emotionally demanding because of the painful confrontation with the child's lost innocence and premature exposure to the uncertain realities of everyday life and the inevitable losses that are part of the life cycle.

This book is a further elaboration of an earlier text, *Children: Stress, Trauma and Disasters,* and a continuing effort to facilitate an understanding of that process to help readers become better able to support children and their families as they cope with and adapt to the traumatic effects of disaster.

Jon A. Shaw, M.D., M.S.

References

Becker-Blease KA, Turner HA, Finkelhor D: Disasters, victimization, and children's mental health. Child Dev 81:1040–1053, 2010

Berkowitz S, Bryant R, Brymer M, et al; National Center for PTSD and the National Child Traumatic Stress Network: Skills for Psychological Recovery: Field Operations Guide. Washington, DC, National Center for PTSD and National Child Traumatic Stress Network, 2010

Copeland WE, Keeler G, Angold A, et al: Traumatic events and posttraumatic stress in childhood. Arch Gen Psychiatry 64:577–584, 2007

Flynn BW: Meeting the needs of special populations in disasters and emergencies: making it work in rural areas. Paper presented at the annual meeting of the National Association for Rural Mental Health, San Antonio, TX, August 2006

National Child Traumatic Stress Network and National Center for PTSD: Psychological First Aid Field Operations Guide, 2nd Edition. 2006. Available at: www.nctsn.org/content/psychological-first-aid. Accessed August 16, 2011.

National Commission on Children and Disasters: 2010 Report to the President and Congress (AHRQ Publ No 10-M037). Rockville, MD, Agency for Healthcare Research and Quality, 2010. Available at: http://archive.ahrq.gov/prep/nccdreport/nccdreport.pdf. Accessed August 16, 2011.

Shultz JM, Espinel Z, Flynn BW, et al: Deep Prep: All-Hazards Disaster Behavioral Health Training. Tampa, FL, Disaster Life Support Publishing, 2007

UNICEF: The State of the World's Children 1997. New York, UNICEF, 1997. Available at: www.unicef.org/sowc97. Accessed August 16, 2011.

UNICEF: Machel Study 10-Year Strategic Review: Children and Conflict in a Changing World. New York, UNICEF, 2009

Acknowledgments

My heartfelt gratitude goes to my many colleagues both in my career as a military psychiatrist and in my academic life who have contributed to my knowledge and understanding of the extraordinary resilience and complexities of the human response to trauma. My fundamental debt is to those survivors of disasters — both personal and otherwise — who have demonstrated so much courage in overcoming adversities and from whom I have learned. My thanks also go to my coauthors, whose rich experiences and thoughtful commentary added to the collaboration, and to John McDuffie and Robert E. Hales of American Psychiatric Publishing for supporting this endeavor and for their timely advice when needed. Also, I want to express my appreciation to my secretary, Michelle Hurtado, whose dedication and persistence resulted in a text, and last but not least to Maria Luisa Urrutia, who understood the time required in such an enterprise and who has been a wonderful companion in our life together.

Jon A. Shaw, M.D., M.S.

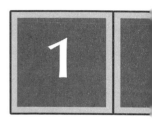

Disaster, Stress, and Trauma

Introduction

Throughout the course of the life cycle, we all are confronted with threats to well-being or even to life itself. Although children are generally exposed to the same spectrum of hazards as adults, they are still maturing physically, emotionally, cognitively, and socially. The impact of perceived threat, psychological trauma, or overt physical harm may become woven into the tapestry of their emergent personalities and their repertoire of adapting and coping capacities. In this chapter, we define terms essential to understanding the psychological effects of trauma exposure: *disaster, stress, primary and secondary stressors, acute and chronic stressors, resilience, traumatic event, acute traumatic moment,* and *traumatic reminders.*

Disaster

Disaster is defined as a severe ecological and psychosocial disruption that greatly exceeds the coping capacity of the community (World Health Organization 1992). Disaster occurs across a timeline that includes preimpact, impact, and postimpact phases (Shaw et al. 2007). During the preimpact phase, community leaders have the opportunity to work with emergency managers to define the range of potential disasters and to develop a comprehensive emergency management plan to provide guidance for the coordination and mobilization of resources in anticipation of the consequences of disasters. The impact phase occurs when the forces of harm impact the community with a likelihood of bodily injury and death and the compromising of community infrastructure and resources. The postimpact phase includes the immediate, intermediate, and subsequent recovery period. Interventions during the postimpact phase are characterized by emergency/rescue efforts and medical/psychosocial interventions to help those affected, to mobilize systems of care, to facilitate resilience, and to address the cascade of secondary adversities such as shortages of food and water, the lack of social supports, economic hardships, and the interruption of utilities and other infrastructure support systems.

Disasters are generally divided into natural or human-generated disasters. *Natural disasters* include weather-related events (hurricanes, tornadoes, and floods), seismic events (earthquakes, tsunamis, and volcanoes), droughts, and pandemics. *Human-generated disasters* are further subdivided into nonintentional versus intentional events (Shultz et al. 2007). Nonintentional human-generated incidents include transportation crashes, hazardous materials spills, and structural collapses reflecting accidental failures of human technologies. In other instances, harm is clearly intended during acts of aggression toward individuals (child maltreatment, assault, rape, and torture) and acts of mass violence (war, civil strife, ethnic conflict, and terrorism). A *mixed,* or *multidimensional, disaster* encompasses elements of both a natural and a human-generated disaster, such as occurred with the 2011 Japanese tsunami and the failure of their nuclear plant safeguards. Disasters, because of their sudden and unpredictable nature, are great sources of stress for the human population.

Stress

Stress is a nonspecific response of the body to any demand placed on the organism. It can be defined as a real or imagined threat to the psychological or physical integrity of the self or as a threat to one's equilibrium or homeostasis. Stress represents an incongruity between the individual's adaptive capacities and the demands placed on the organism (Taylor and Fraser 1981). A child's level of emotional and cognitive development greatly influences his or her psychological response to events in which demands exceed capacities.

It is important to understand the role of subjective appraisal in responding to stress. From a cognitive perspective, stress, like beauty, is often in the eye of the beholder. How one defines a situation determines one's emotional response to it. If a person defines something as real, it is real in its consequences. The same disaster scenario may be perceived by one person as an extremely stressful negative experience but by another person as presenting interesting challenges. As the poet John Milton observed in *Paradise Lost,* "The mind is its own place and in itself, can make a heaven of hell, a hell of heaven." The experience of stress and stressful happenings is an inherent part of the life cycle.

The Spectrum of Stressors

Stressors are events and situations that prompt and provoke the stress response. In this section, we discuss life stressors, contrast primary and secondary stressors, differentiate acute and chronic stressors, and describe distant stressors.

Life Stressors

Life stressors are intrinsic to important milestones in the life cycle. Life/developmental stressors include such events as childbirth, birth of a sibling, early parent death, separation from loved ones, family discord, divorce, aging, hospitalization, surgery, and physical illness. Children who are exposed to such stressors may exhibit clearly discernible behavior changes. For example, a school-age boy who experiences the sudden unexpected death of his father may resume bedwetting, become afraid to sleep alone, and cling to his mother, insisting that he does not want to go to school. Table 1–1 gives examples of stressors in the human experience.

Primary and Secondary Stressors

Primary stressors are associated with acute threats to well-being, physical integrity, and possibly life itself. Primary stressors are associated with direct exposure to the forces of harm during an episode of interpersonal violence or during the period of disaster impact. *Secondary stressors* occur

TABLE 1–1.   **Stressors in the human experience**

| Life/developmental stressors | Disasters and acts of violence | |
	Natural disasters	Human-generated events
Childbirth	Hurricanes	Unintentional events
Birth of a sibling	Tornadoes	Transportation and industrial disasters
Early parent death	Earthquakes	Hazardous materials events
Separation from loved ones	Floods	
	Pandemics	Intentional events
Family discord	Tsunamis	Terrorism
Accidents	Wildfires	War
Financial problems		Civil or ethnic conflict
Divorce		
Hospitalization		Sexual abuse
Surgery		Child maltreatment
Physical illness		Torture
Unemployment		
Aging		

subsequent to a primary stressor as a cluster of consequences or adversities experienced in the aftermath of a traumatic event or disaster. Examples of primary and secondary stressors are noted in Table 1–2. For example, a child who is accidentally burned by scalding water (primary stressor) may experience a multiplicity of secondary stressors, including hospitalization, severe pain, surgical procedures, debridement, scarring and disfigurement, separation from parents, interruption of school attendance, and disruption of daily routines including play activities and socialization.

At the community level, the coastal landfall of a strong hurricane subjects the population in the impact zone to such primary stressors as ravaging winds, storm surge, torrential rainfall, and flooding. The impact phase of the hurricane is circumscribed in time and space. In the storm's aftermath, people in the community experience a cascade of secondary stressors, including disruption of utilities, shortages of basic necessities, damage to homes, displacement, repair delays, loss of valued possessions, school closures, disruption of health care services, unemployment, and economic crisis. Following Hurricane Andrew in 1992, one-quarter of families moved out of the impact zone. Many children discovered that

TABLE 1–2.   **Examples of primary and secondary stressors**

Primary	Secondary
Scalding	Hospitalization
	Surgery
	Debridement
	Separation from parents
	Loss of routines
Hurricane impact, winds, storm surge, tornadoes, floods	Loss of shelter
	School closure
	Unemployment
	Loss of power
	Gasoline shortage
	Evacuation
	Loss of valued possessions
	Separation from loved ones
Explosion of nuclear reactor	Stigmatization of the area
	Unemployment
	Loss of community
	Closing of businesses and schools
	Evacuation
	Fear of cancer risk

their schools were closed and some of their closest friends had moved away (Shaw et al. 1995). Similarly, in 2005, Hurricane Katrina was associated with massive displacement and out-migration from New Orleans. During the 2011 Japanese tsunami and radiation crisis, the government mandated evacuation of the population within a 20-kilometer radius of the damaged nuclear plant.

Acute Versus Chronic Stressors

An *acute stressor* refers to an event that is circumscribed in time and space. The ground-shaking of an earthquake, the touchdown of a tornado, the sudden onslaught of a tsunami, a terrorist attack, and the violence of a physical assault are all examples of acute stressors. Each has a well-defined onset and endpoint. The detonation of the truck bomb that precipitously destroyed the Alfred P. Murrah Federal Building in Oklahoma City in

1995 exemplifies an acute stressor. Forty percent of middle school and high school students in Oklahoma City knew someone who was injured, and one-third knew someone who was killed (Pfefferbaum et al. 1999).

A *chronic stressor* is characterized by ongoing exposure to continuous and unrelenting adversities, such as child maltreatment, war-related trauma, and kidnapping, or to episodic repetitive exposures such as occur with periodic terrorist attacks. Children exposed to chronic stressors may experience a gradual loss of resilience and adaptive coping skills. Cumulative stress is associated with both immediate and long-term neurobiological changes (Cooper et al. 2007), as noted below in the subsection "Chronic Stress Response." Examples of acute and chronic stressors are noted in Table 1–3.

Distant Stressors

A *distant stressor* refers to a traumatic stimulus experienced from a remote and physically safe distance away from the impact zone. A distant stressor may be encountered repetitively through the media or interpersonal interactions. Television networks repeatedly displayed graphic images of the explosive destruction of the space shuttle *Challenger* in 1986, the Oklahoma City bombing in 1995, and the crashing of civilian airliners into the World Trade Center towers on September 11, 2001. These traumatic stimuli were viewed time and time again by children throughout the United States and around the globe. A structured interview that was conducted with children who had viewed the Challenger explosion on television found that 60% experienced specific fears related to death, fires, airplanes, and taking risks (Terr et al. 1999). Sixteen percent of children geographically distant from the Oklahoma City bombing experienced significant posttraumatic stress symptomatology secondary to media exposure (Pfefferbaum et al. 2000). A national survey conducted 3–5 days after the 9/11 attacks revealed that children watched an average of 3 hours of television coverage of the event. One-third of the children had stress symptoms, and 47% were concerned about their own safety (Schuster et al. 2001). In January 2010, televised images of the catastrophic Haiti earthquake were viewed by Miami-based Haitian Americans separated by ocean and 600 miles from the danger zone.

The Stress Response

Acute Stress Response

Direct exposure to a stressor activates the acute stress response, a state of physiological *hyperarousal* frequently described as the fight, flight, or

TABLE 1–3. **Examples of acute and chronic stressors**

	Acute stressors	Chronic stressors
Life/developmental stressors	Motor vehicle accident Surgery Acute illness	Family discord Prolonged separation from loved ones Chronic illness
Natural disasters	Earthquake Hurricane Tornado	Pandemic
Human-generated acts of violence	Single terrorist attack Rape Mugging	War Torture Child maltreatment

freeze response. Encountering a stressor disturbs the body's biological and psychological equilibrium. The stressor is interpreted as potentially threatening to the well-being of the organism.

With the perceived threat, the stress response system in the hypothalamus and brain stem is instantaneously activated. Corticotropin-releasing hormone and arginine vasopressin are secreted by cells in the periventricular region. These neuropeptides are circulated through the vascular system to the anterior part of the pituitary gland, where they stimulate the release of adrenocorticotropic hormone. This hormone stimulates the endocrine system and the adrenal cortex, which produces cortisol. Cortisol has essential and beneficial effects in the short term because it restores depleted energy by increasing glucose availability (Gunnar 2007).

This alarm reaction simultaneously stimulates cells within a region of the brain stem called the *locus coeruleus* (the norepinephrine system), a system that regulates vigilance and fear responses. Through a direct connection with the adrenal medulla, the inner part of the adrenal glands, epinephrine (adrenaline) is released, preparing the individual for a fight-or-flight response (Gunnar 2007). The surge of epinephrine increases heart rate, blood pressure, and respiration, and is accompanied by a sharp spike in glucose, which is released into the bloodstream as an energy source, priming the body for rapid action. Simultaneously, quantities of endorphins, the body's natural painkillers, are secreted. Thus, the short-term response to acute stress involves activation of the hypothalamic-pituitary-adrenal (HPA) axis, secretion of glucocorticoids (cortisol), and activation of the sympathetic nervous system and the release of catecholamines into the circulatory system, enhancing the stress response system and promoting adaptation. Common signs of acute stress are pounding heart, trembling, sweating, shortness of breath, nausea, dizziness, difficulty concentrating, and other vague bodily symptoms.

This adaptive response acts to restore the individual to a more optimal level of function. Regardless of whether the stressor is a minor daily hassle, the so-called common cold, a motor vehicle accident, or an overt threat to life, the human body responds in an attempt to restore order and homeostasis. With sufficient infusion of resources and the passage of time, recovery is the expected outcome of an encounter with an acute stressor (Watson and Shalev 2005).

Chronic Stress Response

Ongoing exposure to chronic stressors usually leads to low cortisol, suggesting adaptation. In some instances, however, the stress response system remains in overdrive, as in the acute stress response, and high levels of epinephrine and cortisol are continuously released. Maintaining the stress response on high alert, however, leads to wear and tear on organ systems and increases the risk for a number of psychobiological symptoms. These include anxiety, depressed mood, sleep and appetite disturbances, interpersonal and social problems, and diminished performance at either school or work. Bodily symptoms such as gastric ulcers, headaches, or irritable bowel syndrome may ensue. When stress and physiological hyperarousal continue unabated, cortisol remains elevated, with possible detrimental effects on immune function and increased risk for chronic conditions such as cardiovascular disease, obesity, depression, hyperthyroidism, diabetes, and even anatomical changes in the brain (McEwen 2004).

In rare instances, the individual's stress response is insufficient to meet the crisis. An inadequate neuroendocrine response with insufficient production of adrenal stress response hormones and cortisol elevates the risk for fibromyalgia, hypothyroidism, or chronic fatigue syndrome (McEwen 2004).

Psychobiological Responses to Chronic Stress in Children

Exposure to ongoing and repetitive traumatic experiences may cause an individual to have profound and reverberating effects, which impact developing neurobiological structures, adaptive and coping strategies, psychological symptom patterns, and even psychopathology. Estimates suggest that up to 80% of children who experience chronic stress (e.g., child victims of aggression and maltreatment by caretakers) will exhibit one or more stress-related disturbances (Bayer et al. 2007; Kendall-Tackett et al. 1993). When children remain suspended in a constant state of fearful expectation, their capacities to use cognitive, social, and emotional experiences to develop solutions to problems are impaired. Continuing exposure to stress may lead to a number of emotional, behavioral, and somatic reactions.

- **Disturbances of behavioral controls** may appear as impulsivity, hyperactivity, aggression, sleep and appetite disturbances, eating disorders, oppositional behavior, substance abuse, and suicidal behaviors.
- **Disturbances in interpersonal relationships** may manifest as social estrangement, interpersonal and family conflicts, problems with boundaries, distrust of others, a belief that intimate relations are dangerous, and avoidance of intimacy.
- **Negative self-attributions** may occur in which the child engages in self-recriminations. Negative self-judgments regarding self-efficacy, competency, and self-worth are paramount and are often associated with a readiness for self-blame, shame, guilt, feelings of helplessness, and self-loathing.
- **Affect dysregulation** may be manifested by irritability, depression, anxiety, mood swings, emotional instability (rage, anger, and despair), suicidal behaviors, hyperarousal, agitation, and substance abuse. Children may experience difficulties in identifying and describing emotions or even knowing what they feel.
- **Disturbances in cognition** may appear as inattention, learning difficulties, problems with information processing, distorted social judgment, alteration in one's systems of meaning (*Weltanschauung*), and an inability to interpret the intentions of others. Other disturbances in thinking are evidenced in memory deficits, denial, repression, suppression, minimization, amnesia, and academic difficulties.
- **Emotional and behavioral problems** may include posttraumatic stress symptoms, mood and other anxiety symptoms, dissociative responses, and severe personality disturbances.

The psychobiological correlates of exposure to chronic stress are directly related to the intensity, duration, and degree of impact of stressors on bodily integrity, the stress response system, and physiological systems critical for sustaining life. The more prolonged the maltreatment, the greater the residual effects. Exposure to intense acute and chronic stressors during the developmental years has enduring neurobiological effects on the stress response, neurotransmitter systems, and anatomical structures. Children who have been physically and sexually abused have decreased brain volumes (decreased size of the cerebrum and the corpus callosum) and poor regulation of the stress response (De Bellis et al. 1999a, 1999b).

Resilience

Resilience is an important mediator of the psychological response to stress, as we discuss further in Chapter 4, "Children's Psychological Responses to Disasters," and Chapter 8, "Interventions." Resilience is a measure of the individual's capacity to rapidly restore predisaster levels of function and psychological equilibrium. Factors that enhance child resilience are effective parenting, positive self-concept, self-regulation, social competence, cognitive flexibility, adaptability to new situations, problem-solving skills, ease with transitions, communication skills, empathy, assertiveness in one's self-interest, humor, religious affiliation, and the ability to elicit caretaking behaviors (Masten 2007).

Trauma
The Traumatic Event

A traumatic event occurs when an individual experiences, witnesses, or is confronted with an event in which there is "actual or threatened death or serious injury, or a threat to the physical integrity of self or others," and when the person's response is associated with "intense fear, helplessness, or horror" (American Psychiatric Association 2000, p. 467). Exposure to trauma may occur from direct physical impact or from directly witnessing harm visually, via media presentation, or through interpersonal relationships with disaster survivors. Experiencing multiple types of trauma exposure increases the risk of psychological consequences.

The essence of the traumatic situation is embodied in feelings of helplessness and fears of imminent death (Shaw 1987). The traumatic event unmasks the illusion of safety and challenges cherished childhood beliefs, such as "Good triumphs over evil," "My parents can always protect me," and "I am invulnerable to injury and death" (Shaw 1987). The individual grapples with the need to accept and cognitively assimilate and integrate the meaning of the experience into his or her conceptual understanding of how the world works and the problem of why bad things happen to good people. The adolescent may be left with a sense of a foreshortened future and take flight into pleasure-seeking or risk-taking activities or, conversely, into a narrowing of the scope of life, phobic inhibitions, or social withdrawal.

Trauma invariably impacts not only the individual but also the family and social system within which the individual lives. The impact of trauma for a child is modulated by the fact that the child has limited life experience. The child is still developing cognitively and emotionally and is often struggling with such issues as separation, individuation, identity formation, and the internalization of predictable mechanisms for regulating intense affects and impulses. Children typically exhibit immature adaptive and coping strategies. When exposed to trauma, children rarely have the capacity to identify emotions such as fear and helplessness and may respond with disorganized or agitated behavior.

The *acute traumatic moment* is defined as the sudden, conscious awareness of vulnerability in the presence of imminent physical injury or death. For children, the sudden awareness that parents are unable to protect and provide for them in their hour of need often ushers in and exacerbates the traumatic moment. The illusion of safety is shattered. The traumatic moment may be associated with feelings of helplessness and anxiety (Shaw 1987).

A distinguishing feature of the traumatic moment is the central role of anxiety and its management. Most commonly, the brief traumatic moment, with its experience of anxiety and helplessness, is followed by rapid remobilization and reintegration of developmentally appropriate coping and adaptive strategies. The child who is able to successfully adapt will restore normal developmental progression with age-appropriate self-direction, academic performance, and peer and family relations. In some instances, distress persists and a failure of reparative defenses leads to a sustained traumatic experience. This may precipitate various degrees of regression with loss of developmental achievements and psychosocial gains as well as various symptoms of somatic ills, anxiety, and mood and behavioral disturbances (Shaw 2000).

Traumatic Reminders

In the aftermath of an acute trauma, the survivor may experience *flashbacks,* in which he or she vividly relives the traumatic moment over and over again. Flashbacks are frequently triggered by *traumatic reminders*, which are external or internal cues that suddenly make the individual feel that the traumatic event is happening again. For example, the sudden and unexpected exposure to strong winds, torrential rains, thunder, and lightning may bring back all the emotions, fears, and cognitions associated with living through a hurricane. A child who was once painfully injured in a bicycle accident may reexperience all the emotions, ideations, and physical sensations of that event when exposed to the cue of seeing another child's mangled bicycle.

Cumulative Risk

The philosopher Friedrich Nietzsche wrote, "That which does not kill us makes us stronger," indicating that perhaps trauma exposure has an inoculating or protective effect for subsequent trauma exposure. Little evidence supports this point of view. Instead, the general evidence indicates that as the number of traumatic events experienced accumulates, an individual has an increasing risk of subsequent emotional and behavioral problems and negative adaptation. A *dose-response effect* occurs, in that with increased frequency of exposure to multiple traumatic events, a child is more likely to experience posttraumatic stress symptomatology. Catani et al. (2010) demonstrated that children exposed to a tsunami, war-related trauma, and family violence suffered from the cumulative effect of trauma exposure and therefore suffered more psychosocial adjustment and poorer adaptation than children not exposed to all three types of traumatic life events. Chemtob et al. (2008) found that conjoined exposure to the 9/11 attacks and other traumatic events increased the risk for behavioral problems in children. Garrison et al. (1993) assessed 1,264 children ages 11–17 years and found that survivors of Hurricane Hugo who had a previous exposure to violent traumatic events were more likely to develop posttraumatic stress disorder.

■ Key Clinical Points

- ■ Children and adolescents are exposed to various types of stress and traumatic events during their developmental years.

- ■ Primary or acute stressors are relatively circumscribed in time and space.

■ Secondary stressors are invariably present in the postimpact and recovery phases.

■ A traumatic event occurs when an individual experiences, witnesses, or is confronted with a situation in which there is a perceived or real threat of bodily injury or a threat to life itself.

■ The acute traumatic moment for children is frequently ushered in by the discovery that parents are not able to protect them and the sudden awareness of vulnerability in the presence of imminent physical injury or death.

■ The individual response to stress is shaped by the impact of the fateful event and by one's subjective appraisal.

■ Individuals have a psychobiological response to acute and chronically occurring stressors.

■ Resilience is an important mediator of the response to stress.

■ Traumatic reminders refer to events in the aftermath of traumatic exposure that cause the child or adolescent to relive and reexperience the trauma as if it were occurring once again.

■ Multiple trauma exposures combine in a dose-response manner and increase the risk for psychological morbidity.

References

American Psychiatric Association: Diagnostic and Statistical Manual of Mental Disorders, 4th Edition, Text Revision. Washington, DC, American Psychiatric Association, 2000

Bayer CP, Klasen F, Adam H: Association of trauma and PTSD symptoms with openness to reconciliation and feelings of revenge among former Ugandan and Congolese child soldiers. JAMA 298:555–559, 2007

Catani C, Gewirtz AH, Weiling E, et al: Tsunami, war and cumulative risk in the lives of Sri Lankan schoolchildren. Child Dev 81:1176–1191, 2010

Chemtob CM, Nomura Y, Abramovitz RA: Impact of conjoined exposure to the World Trade Center attacks and to other traumatic events on the behavior problems of preschool children. Arch Pediatr Adolesc Med 162:126–133, 2008

Cooper NS, Feder A, Southwick AM, et al: Resiliency and vulnerability to trauma, in Adolescent Psychopathology and the Developing Brain. Edited by Romer D, Walker EF. Oxford, UK, Oxford University Press, 2007, pp 347–372

De Bellis MD, Baum AS, Birmaher B, et al: A.E. Bennett Research Award. Developmental traumatology, part I: biological stress systems. Biol Psychiatry 45:1259–1270, 1999a

De Bellis MD, Keshavan MS, Clark DB, et al: A.E. Bennett Research Award. Developmental traumatology, part II: brain development. Biol Psychiatry 45:1271–1284, 1999b

Garrison CZ, Weinrich MW, Hardin SB, et al: Post-traumatic stress disorder in adolescents after a hurricane. Am J Epidemiol 138:522–530, 1993

Gunnar MR: Stress effects on the developing brain, in Adolescent Psychopathology and the Developing Brain. Edited by Romer D, Walker EF. Oxford, UK, Oxford University Press, 2007, pp 127–147

Kendall-Tackett KA, Williams LM, Finkelhor D: Impact of sexual abuse on children: a review and synthesis of recent empirical studies. Psychol Bull 113:164–180, 1993

Masten A: Competence, resilience and development, in Adolescent Psychopathology and the Developing Brain. Edited by Romer D, Walker EF. Oxford, UK, Oxford University Press, 2007, pp 31–52

McEwen B: Protective and damaging effects of stress mediators. Seminars in Medicine of the Beth Israel Deaconess Medical Center 338:171–179, 2004

Pfefferbaum B, Nixon SJ, Krug RS, et al: Clinical needs assessment of middle and high school students following the 1995 Oklahoma City bombing. Am J Psychiatry 156:1069–1074, 1999

Pfefferbaum B, Seale TW, McDonald NB, et al: Posttraumatic stress two years after the Oklahoma City bombing in youths geographically distant from the explosion. Psychiatry 63:358–370, 2000

Schuster MA, Stein BD, Jaycox L, et al: A national survey of stress reactions after the September 11, 2001, terrorist attacks. N Engl J Med 345:1507–1512, 2001

Shaw JA: Unmasking of the illusion of safety: psychic trauma in war. Bull Menninger Clin 51:49–63, 1987

Shaw JA: Children, adolescents and trauma. Psychiatr Q 71:227–243, 2000

Shaw JA, Applegate B, Tanner S, et al: Psychological effects of Hurricane Andrew on an elementary school population. J Am Acad Child Adolesc Psychiatry 34:1185–1192, 1995

Shaw JA, Espinel Z, Shultz JM: Children: Stress, Trauma and Disasters. Tampa, FL, Disaster Life Support Publishing, 2007

Shultz JM, Espinel Z, Flynn BW, et al: Deep Prep: All-Hazards Disaster Behavioral Health Training. Tampa, FL, Disaster Life Support Publishing, 2007

Taylor AJW, Fraser AG: Psychological Sequelae of Operation Overdue Following the DC-10 Aircrash in Antarctica (Victoria University of Wellington Publications in Psychology No 27) Wellington, New Zealand, Victoria University, 1981

Terr LC, Bloch DA, Michel BA, et al: Children's symptoms in the wake of Challenger: a field study of distant-traumatic effects and an outline of related conditions. Am J Psychiatry 156:1536–1544, 1999

Watson PJ, Shalev AY: Assessment and treatment of adult acute responses to traumatic stress following mass traumatic events. CNS Spectr 10:123–131, 2005

World Health Organization, Division of Mental Health: Psychosocial Consequences of Disaster: Prevention and Management. Geneva, World Health Organization, 1992

2

Natural and Human-Generated Disasters

Introduction

"The stars are against us" is the interpretation that derives from melding the Latin root words *dis* and *astrum* to create the word *disaster*. The World Health Organization (1992) defined *disaster* as a severe ecological and psychosocial disruption that greatly exceeds the coping capacity of the altered community. We use a parallel but expanded definition: "A disaster is characterized as an encounter between forces of harm and a human population in harm's way, influenced by the ecological context, in which the demands of the situation exceed the coping capacity of the affected population" (Shaw et al. 2007, p. 23). The common theme that unifies these definitions is disproportionate demand on the population. A disaster overwhelms the community's resources at many levels, including the abilities of children and families to cope psychologically.

The scope and scale of urgent events can be described using terms that represent a hierarchy of demand: *crisis, emergency, disaster, catastrophe,* and *complex emergency* (Quarantelli 2006; Toole 1990).

1. In a *crisis* situation, the community has ample intrinsic resources to manage the situation.
2. An *emergency* is more challenging, but local assets are still able to manage the needs.
3. A *disaster* occurs when demand exceeds coping capacity, requiring a call for outside assistance.
4. A *catastrophe* is a disaster so extreme that the community's capability to respond is essentially obliterated.
5. A *complex emergency* is a severe psychosocial disruption often characterized by war and civil confict and loss of food and logistical support systems that frequently results in population displacement and refugees.

The devastation wrought upon the city of New Orleans by Hurricane Katrina graphically depicts a catastrophe. On the morning of August 29, 2005, a Category 3 hurricane made landfall just east of New Orleans. On that same day, two major levees protecting the city were breached. By the morning of August 30, about 8% of New Orleans was under water, stranding 50,000–100,000 citizens, with many clinging to rooftops. More than 25,000 people sought shelter in the New Orleans Superdome. City and regional support services were submerged in floodwaters and inoperable. Food, water, and electrical power, as well as emergency and life-support services, were unavailable or inaccessible. Community infrastructure was destroyed, looting was widespread, and political and ethnic fissures quickly surfaced with allegations of blame and racism. Reflecting on Katrina, Quarantelli (2006) described the elements that make a catastrophe categorically distinct from a disaster: 1) emergency organizations and operational bases are so severely strained that they become unresponsive; 2) city and local officials are unable to perform their leadership roles; 3) community services are destroyed, and assistance from the affected community is not available; 4) local mass media ceases to function, and so the disaster is described by news sources from afar; and 5) conflict surfaces along the fault lines of race, class, and ethnicity.

Other examples of catastrophes that became major complex emergencies include the 2004 Southeast Asia tsunami and the 2010 Haiti earthquake.

Disaster Classification

Disasters are generally divided into two broad categories: *natural disasters* and *human-generated disasters*. There is increasing recognition of a third category, *multidimensional disaster,* which encompasses both an act of nature and a nonintentional human-generated disaster. When a multidimensional disaster evolves into a major humanitarian crisis, it can be considered a *complex emergency.* A classification of disasters is presented in Table 2–1.

Natural Disasters

Natural disasters are described as *acts of nature.* As shown in Table 2–1, natural disasters are subcategorized as meteorological, hydrological, geophysical, climatological, or biological.

Direct or vicarious exposure to natural disasters is part of the life experience of the majority of individuals. Most persons are familiar with a variety of natural disasters and recognize their relatively common occurrence. Although risks and types of natural disasters vary by region, data from studies conducted throughout the United States suggest that approximately 10%–20% of people will experience direct exposure to a natural disaster during their lifetime (Breslau et al. 1998; Copeland et al. 2007; Kessler et al. 1995). Although mitigation strategies may diminish the severity of impact, most natural disasters are not preventable.

A longitudinal study of children in western North Carolina indicated that 11% had been exposed to a natural disaster before age 16 years (Copeland et al. 2007). Similarly, in a survey of 2,030 U.S. children, ages 2–17 years, lifetime exposure to a natural disaster was found to be 13.9%, with 4.1% of survey participants reporting exposure within the past year (Becker-Blease et al. 2010). For those reporting experience with a disaster, 27% indicated that they had been in a tornado, 24% reported exposure to a hurricane, and 18% had directly experienced an earthquake.

Human-Generated Disasters

Human-generated disasters are usually *nonintentional* and most typically involve a failure of human technology. Examples include transportation accidents (air and rail crashes), structural collapses (buildings, tunnels, bridges, stadiums), industrial accidents, and releases of hazardous materials (liquid spills, aerosolized chemical or radiation leaks). Other

TABLE 2–1.   Classification of disaster

Natural disasters
Meteorological (weather-related) disasters
   Tropical cyclones (hurricanes, cyclones, typhoons, tropical storms)
   Tornadoes
   Storms (thunderstorms, winter storms)
Hydrological disasters (floods and related disasters)
   Floods
   Landslides/mudslides
   Avalanches
Geophysical disasters
   Earthquakes
   Volcanic eruptions
   Tsunamis
Climatological disasters
   Extreme temperatures
   Wildfires
   Droughts
Biological disasters
   Pandemic diseases
   Crop blights
   Diseases of domesticated animals

Human-generated disasters
Nonintentional/technological
   Industrial accidents
   Transportation accidents
   Ecological/environmental destruction
   Miscellaneous accidents
Intentional
   Declared war
   Civil strife
   Ethnic conflict
   Violent mass gatherings and demonstrations
   Terrorism

Complex emergencies
Extensive violence, loss of life, displacement, societal/economic
   disruption
Need for large-scale, multifaceted humanitarian assistance

forms of human-generated disasters may create ecological or environmental destruction. Failures of technology that result in disaster are rarely intentional, although poor judgment and negligence may be relevant human factors in determining the degree of psychological impact.

In contrast to technological disasters, episodes of war, civil strife, ethnic violence, and terrorism may result in *intentional* perpetration of harm. Unlike exposure to natural disasters, direct exposure to human-generated acts of violence tends to be outside common experience, unfamiliar, unanticipated, and unpredictable (Institute of Medicine 2003). Purposeful intent to do harm characterizes both interpersonal aggression at the individual level (Breslau et al. 1998) and acts of mass violence at the community level. Survivors of intentional acts of violence are at elevated risk for severe psychological morbidity compared with individuals who experience either natural disasters or nonintentional human-generated events (Norris et al. 2002).

Multidimensional Disasters

A multidimensional disaster combines the features of both natural and human-generated nonintentional disasters. For example, in 2005, the landfall of Hurricane Katrina (natural disaster) precipitated the breaching of the levees surrounding New Orleans (a human construction); these hazards combined to amplify the damage, destruction, mortality, and trauma associated with this event. In 2011, an earthquake measuring magnitude 9.0 on the Richter scale occurred off the east coast of Japan and generated a tsunami (natural event), the runup of which overtopped the seawalls protecting several nuclear power plants. The reactor cooling systems were damaged, leading to partial meltdown and radiation releases (human-generated event) over populated areas.

A schema for disaster classification is presented in Figure 2–1.

Disaster Life Cycle

A disaster progresses through specific phases across a timeline. At the most basic level of conceptualization, the timeline is divided into preimpact, impact, and postimpact phases.

Preimpact Phase

The preimpact phase includes the period between disasters when disaster planning is conducted, hazard mitigation programs are implemented,

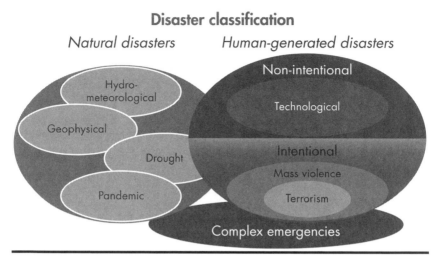

Disaster classification

Natural disasters   *Human-generated disasters*

FIGURE 2–1.   **Disaster classification.**
Source.   Shultz et al. 2007.

and citizen participation in disaster preparedness is encouraged. For example, a coastal community can confront hurricane hazards by strengthening building codes, installing hurricane shutters, devising evacuation plans, constructing water management/flood mitigation systems to minimize inland flooding, and recruiting citizens to join neighborhood emergency response teams.

The preimpact phase also includes the period when a disaster threat is detected and warnings are issued, alerting the public that a disaster is probable or imminent. Flood, tornado, hurricane, and tsunami warnings are issued in the areas where a strike is most likely. Credible intelligence regarding a terrorist threat may prompt the federal government to raise the alert level and notify the public of actions to take. The mental health significance for children and families is that any actions that can be taken to dampen the destructiveness of disaster hazards and to separate citizens from direct encounter with harmful forces will reduce trauma and psychological consequences related to the event.

Impact Phase

During the impact phase, citizens may experience the full fury of the forces of harm. This phase is associated with the maximum likelihood of bodily injury and death, physical destruction, and widespread community disruption. Individuals in harm's way often fear for their lives, and they may witness scenes of devastation or extreme harm to others. Some survivors will sustain injury, whereas others may lose a loved one through disaster-related death. Children may lose a parent or primary caregiver. Invariably, survivors in the disaster-affected community will know someone who was injured or killed in a disaster, and this experience is likely to produce varying degrees of emotional distress. Pfefferbaum et al. (2001) surveyed 2,000 middle-school children 7 weeks after the 1995 Oklahoma City bombing and found that 50% knew someone who had been either killed or injured. The level of psychiatric risk varies with the specific nature of the disaster, the degree of personal exposure, the extent of physical destruction and community disruption, and the range of stressful adversities in the aftermath.

Confronted by overwhelming forces during disaster impact, both children and adults may experience a sense of helplessness. A profound feeling of helplessness is the essence of the traumatic situation.

Some individuals respond to the urgent demands of an ongoing disaster event with heroic efforts to save themselves, family members, neighbors, and community assets. Often, survivors come together with a renewed sense of group cohesiveness and solidarity in an effort to protect the community and to mobilize resources for recovery. Immediately after the danger subsides, a profound sense of relief and triumph often emerges for those individuals who have escaped injury and death and are able to reunite with loved ones who have also survived.

Postimpact Phase

Following the impact of a disaster, survivors may enter a prolonged period of cascading secondary adversities. In this postimpact phase, a rising tide of disillusionment may emerge as people become aware of the enormity of the tasks necessary to achieve full recovery. Survivors take stock of the inventory of secondary stressors, such as loss of home and shelter, closure of schools, unemployment, economic losses, damage to community infrastructure, loss of social supports, and pervasive psychological distress and impairment. The recovery phase requires survivors to navigate their way through a tangled bureaucratic process. Survivors must negotiate with insurance adjusters, code inspectors, and local, state, and national authorities to acquire the help and the financial assistance that is available to those who persevere. A sobering realization settles over the survivors as they come to understand that recovery is a process that takes years. For many children and families, enduring the postimpact adversities is more challenging than withstanding the forceful assault of the disaster impact itself. The brief, acute, and extreme stressors of impact subside, only to be succeeded by the prolonged, chronic, and debilitating stressors in the aftermath.

The community psychosocial response to disaster is interwoven with the disaster life cycle. Ahearn and Cohen (1985), followed by Zunin and Myers (2000), described a trajectory of community psychosocial response to a major disaster that has been found to broadly apply across a range of disaster types. Zunin and Myers (2000) described the community's progression through the stages of disaster impact, heroism, community solidarity, disillusionment, and reconstruction (Figure 2–2).

This sequence of community response can be applied to the September 11, 2001, attacks on America. As the civilian aircraft slammed into the Twin Towers of the World Trade Center, there was a momentary stun reaction and a period of disbelief, as persons grappled with both the novelty and the terror of the situation. Within moments, however, occupants of the buildings banded together, helping one another to descend the stairwells and find safe passage to the street. Almost all who had an unobstructed escape route were able to exit the buildings safely. Survivors were aided throughout the process by courageous responders and helpful citizens. As part of this brief, life-saving *heroic phase,* individuals who escaped the Twin Towers experienced relief associated with their survival. During the next several days, and extending for a period of weeks, Americans came together with a sense of national resolve and a heightened spirit of patriotism, actions that embody the *community solidarity stage.* They had a unified belief that America would prevail against the terrorists. This outpouring of nationalistic feelings and enhanced sense of revitalization has been described as a stage of euphoria or postdisaster utopia, in which the communal body mobilizes its resources and individuals bind their anxiety by immersing themselves in community with an increasing sense of national solidarity.

As predicted by the models, in subsequent months following 9/11, there was a more protracted *disillusionment stage,* marked by national uncertainty and insecurity, changes in the American lifestyle (such as the implementation of airport security measures), fears of other attacks, emerging disappointments, and a readiness to externalize blame onto political leaders and government officials for not doing enough to protect the nation. Eventually, within the *recovery,* or *reconstruction, stage,* Americans came to accept the *new normal,* a more realistic appraisal of risks and dangers, and proactive changes to protect the American nation and its lifestyle. A few months before the 10-year anniversary of the attack, the tedious and painstaking hunt for Osama bin Laden finally led to his killing, prompting joyous celebration as well as painful remembrance throughout America.

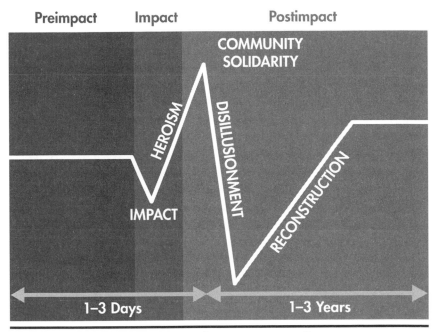

Preimpact   Impact   Postimpact

COMMUNITY SOLIDARITY

HEROISM

DISILLUSIONMENT

IMPACT

RECONSTRUCTION

1–3 Days   1–3 Years

FIGURE 2–2.   Stage of community response to disaster.
Source.   Zunin and Myers 2000.

Common Natural Disasters

Hurricanes

A hurricane is a tropical cyclone, typically hundreds of miles in diameter, characterized by powerful winds, torrential rains, and storm surge. These forces of harm may trigger inland flooding, mudslides, and tornadoes. The eyewall has the most intense cyclonic winds, which rotate ferociously around the perimeter of the calm eye of the storm.

Tropical cyclones form in seven hurricane basins distributed along the midsection of the globe, both north and south of the equator. Tropical cyclones occurring in the Atlantic and Eastern Pacific basins are called *hurricanes.* The number of hurricanes that form annually in each basin is affected by many factors, including ocean temperatures and global weather systems. In the Atlantic basin, the official hurricane season extends from June 1 to November 30, with a sharp peak in August and September. Hurricane frequency rises and falls over 30- to 50-year cycles, and the 2000s thus far represent a period of increased frequency. The current active period for Atlantic basin hurricanes is anticipated to continue for another 10–15 years (Klotzbach and Gray 2005).

Hurricanes are identified and tracked as they move across the ocean waters, often maintaining hurricane strength for hundreds of miles and for periods ranging from hours to weeks. Some storms remain over the open ocean, never affecting island or coastal inhabitants. Other hurricanes make multiple landfalls (in 2004, Hurricane Ivan devastated the island of Grenada before hammering Alabama and the panhandle of Florida, continuing inland to Virginia, and then drifting back into the Atlantic and circling back to cross the Florida peninsula and make landfall again in Louisiana) or track parallel to coastlines, deluging land areas beneath a spiraling canopy of thunderstorms (in 1998, Hurricane Mitch lingered over warm Caribbean waters, just offshore from Honduras, Guatemala, and Nicaragua, as unceasing rains generated a series of deadly mudslides, before eventually making landfall).

The National Hurricane Center (2011) issues a hurricane watch for coastal areas when there is a potential for hurricane landfall within 24–36 hours. A hurricane warning "is issued 48 hours in advance of the anticipated onset of tropical-storm-force winds." Long warning periods provide the opportunity for families to prepare and to evacuate if necessary.

Preimpact Hurricane Stressors

Hurricane watches and warnings provide advance notice to citizens, giving them time to protect property, shutter windows, safeguard family members, and move from harm's way by evacuating inland or relocating to shelters. Nevertheless, hurricane warnings provoke anticipatory anxiety and emotional distress given the uncertainty as to when and where the hurricane will make landfall. Often, a contagion of fear and anxiety spreads as families and the community prepare for the storm. Community members may frantically shop for food, water, flashlights, batteries, generators, and materials such as shutters and plywood for boarding up windows. Long lines may form as cars queue up for gasoline in preparation for evacuation. Acute shortages of supplies commonly occur. Families struggle to consolidate plans to be together in one safe place or to evacuate as an intact family group. Decisions must be made about sheltering in place or selecting essential items for each family member if rapid evacuation is necessary.

Impact Phase Hurricane Stressors

Long before the eye of a hurricane makes landfall, communication networks may become inoperable. Loss of electrical power may jeopardize food and water supplies. While the hurricane is at full force, threats of physical injury and fears for one's life are common as the powerful storm propels wind-driven projectiles, shatters windows, destroys roofs, and creates massive physical destruction over large areas. Tropical storm– and hurricane-force winds may continue for many hours, accompanied by terrifying sounds of shrieking winds and nearby storm destruction, accentuated by palpable changes in air pressure. Driving rains, tornadoes, and inland flooding create additional hazards. During impact, children may observe signs of anxiety and fear in their parents and caretakers, undermining their own sense of safety and their confidence in their parents' abilities to protect them. Eighty-five percent of children who directly experienced the impact of Hurricane Andrew in 1992 manifested moderate to severe levels of posttraumatic stress symptoms (Shaw et al. 1995).

Postimpact Hurricane Stressors

After a storm, children may face major disruptions of normal routines. School closures are common. Damage to their home neighborhoods may be extreme. Community landmarks may be damaged or destroyed. Children may lose favorite toys, valued personal memorabilia, and even beloved pets. Children may experience the horror of seeing severely injured survivors or dead bodies. Twenty-one months following Hurricane Andrew, 70% of the children continued to manifest moderate to severe posttraumatic stress symptoms and many exhibited increasing emotional and behavioral problems related to the multiplicity of secondary adversities (Shaw et al. 1996).

Hurricane Katrina was among the worst natural disasters to impact the United States. There was a mandatory evacuation of the entire city. More than 1,800 lives were lost, including many victims who were drowned inside their homes as surging floodwaters engulfed them. Although the majority of families escaped prior to the collapse of the levees, many of the city's citizens, including the poor, elderly, and children, had no means of evacuating and were forced to seek refuge in their attics or on the roofs of their homes. Large emergency shelters were activated just before landfall in the Superdome and the New Orleans Convention Center. Many children had to wade through floodwaters to safety or endure precarious journeys to a distant point of refuge. Children in New Orleans frequently experienced separation from family members, triggering fear reactions and feelings of desperation.

The major emergency shelters lost electricity, leaving their inhabitants without air conditioning, working toilets, cold water, or hot food during the sweltering days before the people were rescued. Interpersonal violence erupted in the shelters, including reported sexual assaults. Prior to evacuation, many young children and elderly became seriously ill and had to be hospitalized. Because of procedural flaws, many children were separated from family members during the evacuation. Hundreds of families were subsequently evacuated to the Houston Astrodome. Ethnic tensions flared as hurricane-displaced African American children were suddenly inserted into a predominantly Latino community. On the heels of Katrina, Hurricane Rita struck the Gulf Coast on September 24, 2001, delaying the reopening of New Orleans and causing further damage and dislocation.

Upon their eventual return to New Orleans, many families faced an extended stay in cramped, crowded Federal Emergency Management Agency (FEMA) trailers. Some children were relocated multiple times. Anecdotal reports gathered during Project Fleur-de-lis documented the highly stressful conditions. Jamming extended families into temporary trailers exposed many children, at close quarters, to adults consuming alcohol, having sex, and committing acts of aggression and domestic violence (Cohen et al. 2009).

With a sprawling, federally declared disaster area extending across 90,000 square miles of the Gulf of Mexico coastline, Hurricane Katrina was described as the most costly and damaging disaster in U.S. history (Kilmer and Gil-Rivas 2010). Hundreds of people remained missing and more than 1,800 were confirmed dead after the storm (Kessler et al. 2006). As many as 100,000 residents of New Orleans, primarily of minority race and ethnicity, were unable to evacuate from the city (Cordasco et al. 2007). The baseline rate of "any" mental illness doubled from 15% to 30% post-Katrina (Kessler et al. 2006). A study conducted from 18 to 27 months post-Katrina, with a probability sample of children ages 4–17 years, found that 15% met criteria to be classified as seriously emotionally disturbed. When compared with the 5% prestorm baseline rate of serious emotional disturbance (Costello et al. 1998), these findings suggest that approximately 10% of the children who experienced Hurricane Katrina developed serious emotional disturbance that was directly attributable to the effects of disaster exposure (McLaughlin et al. 2009).

The economic costs of the mental health effects of the 2005 Hurricanes Katrina and Rita were estimated based on the assumption that overall psychiatric morbidity peaked at 33% of the direct impact survivors in the first year. Investigators converted this to a per capita cost estimate of $1,133, equivalent to $12.5 billion for the entire affected population (Schoenbaum et al. 2009).

Hurricane Traumatic Reminders

Common traumatic reminders for individuals who have experienced hurricanes are the annual onset of hurricane season, hurricane warnings, the sudden appearance of towering dark clouds, bolts of lightning, torrential rains, gusting winds, and hurricane preparedness activities.

Earthquakes

Abrupt, powerful movements of the earth's crust along tectonic plate boundaries generate the seismic forces that produce earthquakes, sending shock waves laterally, or up and down, over very large surface areas. The earthquake mainshock lasts only seconds, or several minutes at most, and is accompanied by a low-pitched rumbling that resembles the sound of a freight train.

In contrast to hurricanes, earthquakes occur suddenly without warning. More than 20,000 perceptible temblors are estimated to occur annually, with half of these registering at magnitude 5.0 or greater on the Richter scale (Ursano et al. 2009). Annually, only 1 in 300 of these seismic events (about 70 per year) produces a notable earthquake that directly affects a human population. Of these earthquakes, very few (less than one per year) cause catastrophic damage, destruction, injury, and death.

Earthquake strength is measured by two methods. The Richter scale measures the amount of energy released by the earthquake. The surface strength of an earthquake varies from imperceptible to extreme. The Modified Mercalli Intensity Scale measures the amount of damage and destruction caused by the earthquake and is a preferred metric for estimating human impact. The scale ranges from level I (not felt) to level XII (total destruction). The 2010 Haiti earthquake, measuring 7.0 on the Richter scale, demonstrated the enormous destructive potential of an earthquake. The quake caused an estimated 222,570 deaths and 300,000 injuries requiring medical attention. Almost 1 in 5 Haitians were displaced, with 1.3 million moving to improvised camps in the immediate vicinity of destruction and 600,000 relocating to remote rural areas of the country. The earthquake was ranked level X (extreme) on the Mercalli scale. More recently, on March 11, 2011, the fourth strongest earthquake in the world since 1900, measuring 9.0 on the Richter scale, occurred off the east coast of Japan and launched a major tsunami with devastating consequences; a wall of water mounting 10 meters in amplitude destroyed coastal cities.

Earthquakes may destroy government and commercial buildings, schools, homes, bridges, dams, and highways. Severed gas mains and downed power lines may ignite fires, and disruption of water supplies and buckled roadways may interfere with the firefighting response. Water supplies may become contaminated from broken sewage lines, increasing the risk for infectious diseases. Unpredictable aftershocks occur frequently for days to months afterward, sometimes causing more damage and injury than the original quake. Aftershocks also serve as powerful trauma reminders of the initial mainshock.

Earthquakes originating beneath the ocean's floor may generate a tsunami (from the Japanese words *tsu* for harbor and *nami* for wave), enormous waves moving outward from the epicenter with extraordinary velocity and propulsion. The great Sumatra-Andaman earthquake of December 26, 2004, produced an Indian Ocean tsunami that resulted in 283,000 deaths along thousands of miles of coastline, with the highest recorded death tolls occurring in Indonesia, India, Sri Lanka, and Thailand. This tsunami rapidly evolved into a humanitarian crisis characterized by mass bereavement and displacement of more than 1 million persons (Lay et al. 2005). A study of 325 tsunami-exposed adolescents in Sri Lanka found that mediators of postdisaster mental health included the intensity of traumatic exposure, displacement from home, loss of social and family supports, and maternal depression (Wickrama and Kaspar 2007). Conversely, a positive mother-child relationship was a protective factor that diminished the rate and severity of depressive and posttraumatic stress symptoms in the adolescents.

Preimpact Earthquake Stressors

The reality that significant earthquakes occur rarely and unpredictably may breed complacency. Persons living in seismically active areas may minimize or distort the objective reality of earthquake risk. However, disaster-savvy families can mitigate this risk by locating away from tectonic plate boundary zones and other areas of extreme earthquake risk. Other options include selecting new, well-constructed housing that conforms to earthquake building codes, or retrofitting and disaster proofing older housing units. Involving the family in the creation of an all-hazards family disaster plan that includes periodic earthquake drills is a prudent strategy.

Impact and Postimpact Earthquake Stressors

The sudden, unexpected, and violent experience of the ground shaking during an earthquake may provoke feelings of helplessness, terror, and fear. In fact, this subjective experience of forceful ground shaking, especially when accompanied by perceived threat to life, is one of the strongest predictors of posttraumatic stress symptoms for earthquake survivors (Basoglu et al. 2009). The earth's apparent stability is instantaneously transformed into a landscape of quaking destruction. Individuals and families may be injured and trapped in collapsed structures when homes, schools, shopping centers, and highways succumb to the shaking forces that may actually cause liquefaction of the earth close to the quake's center. The ground literally loses its weight-bearing capacity and emulsifies, causing structures to sink and disintegrate.

Children exposed to the 1988 Armenia earthquake displayed increased rates of posttraumatic stress disorder (PTSD), and adolescents exhibited altered neurohormonal stress responses 5 years after exposure (Pynoos et al. 1998). A study of 2,037 children, ages 9–17 years, who were exposed to the 1999 Athens earthquake found that PTSD rates were highest for those who were directly impacted and those with the highest degree of perceived threat (Giannopoulou et al. 2006). PTSD rates were higher for younger children and for girls. The strongest predictor of depression was the degree of postearthquake adversity.

During an earthquake, children may witness grotesque scenes of severe injury, entrapment, crushed bodies, and brutal death. Widespread harm and ongoing danger may be compounded by the abrupt loss of community infrastructure, power and other utilities, communications systems, and health care services. Obtaining basic necessities such as food and water may become an acute challenge.

Children may become separated from parents and family members during an earthquake, and hours or days may pass before they know whether their loved ones are safe. Far more agonizing, in the case of great tsunamis, the bodies of thousands of persons who are caught by the waves are washed out to sea and many never reappear. Surviving family members may assume that their loved ones have perished but they have proof of neither life nor death. For these survivors, and especially for children, uncertainty and lack of closure amplify the distress of bereavement.

For children exposed to the 1994 Northridge earthquake in Los Angeles, the risk for posttraumatic stress symptoms was related to the degree of life threat, the frequency of exposure to trauma reminders such as aftershocks and signs of physical damage to their dwelling, and their subjective appraisal of their own actions during the earthquake (Pynoos et al. 1998). Epidemiological analyses of earthquake survivors in Turkey and Greece consistently documented that fear during the earthquake and perceived life threat were significant predictors of psychological distress and PTSD (Basoglu et al. 2009; Sumer et al. 2005).

Injuries are common in earthquakes, particularly because of the abrupt, cataclysmic collapse of structures. The most common injuries are fractures and dislocations, and various head, face, and brain injuries. Many survivors are buried under the rubble and may be entrapped, often with delayed rescue. This experience may lead to severe trauma to extremities, and amputating injuries are common. An injured child may require ongoing and protracted medical intervention and pain management; the experience of medical treatment and rehabilitation is itself a secondary stressor.

Earthquake Traumatic Reminders

Sudden and repetitive earthquake aftershocks intensify anxiety and fear responses because they recreate the sensations of the initial quake (Basoglu et al. 2004; Kuwabara et al. 2008; Lau et al. 2010). Traumatic reminders may also include jagged cracks in walls and masonry, rumbling noises, unrepaired and heavily damaged buildings, piles of rubble, strong odors of fire or decay, and broadcast news reports about the earthquake.

Tornadoes

A tornado is a violently rotating column of air, in contact with the ground, beneath a cumuliform cloud, that is typically visible as a funnel cloud (Glickman 2000). The U.S. Midwest experiences the highest frequency of tornadoes in the world and has earned the moniker Tornado Alley. Tornadoes may be up to 2 miles in width at the base, and wind speeds, graded on the Enhanced Fujita Scale, may exceed 200 miles per hour. Tornadoes most commonly occur in the spring and summer, touching down in erratic, jagged, and unpredictable paths. A single storm system may include dozens or even hundreds of tornadoes, described as a tornado family or outbreak. These multiple tornado systems can be particularly deadly, as in the April 25–28, 2011, outbreak that focused on Alabama and affected 20 other states, from Texas to New York; at least 336 separate tornadoes killed an estimated 346 persons, creating the fourth deadliest tornado event in U.S. history.

Tornado-driven devastation is immediate and sporadically extreme; buildings may be explosively destroyed in a matter of seconds. In the United States, approximately 800 tornadoes form during a typical year, collectively causing about 1,500 injuries and 80 deaths.

Preimpact Tornado Stressors

Advances in weather prediction and forecasting have reduced tornado-related injuries and fatalities. Tornado "watch boxes" are posted for areas where climatic conditions are conducive to tornado formation. Neverthe-less, the warning period for active tornadoes is brief under the best cir-cumstances and nonexistent for many areas. When a tornado warning is issued, families must take shelter immediately. The period of warning and rapid sheltering is stressful for millions of persons each tornado sea-son, with thousands of warnings issued by the National Weather Service nationwide.

Impact and Postimpact Tornado Stressors

Single tornadoes do not typically create widespread destruction on the scale of hurricane damage. Damage patterns tend to be spotty and in-consistent, with areas of complete devastation interspersed with areas that are untouched. Intense tornadoes produce extreme pressure gradi-ents that may shatter buildings in the path of destruction. Alternatively, entire structures such as houses, barns, and silos have been lifted from their foundations and hurled airborne for great distances. In May 2007, a devastating 1.7-mile-wide tornado destroyed 95% of all dwellings and structures in Greensburg, Kansas.

Children may see collapsed buildings, destroyed barns, and dead farm animals, and experience the horror of seeing severely injured peo-ple or dead bodies. The sudden onset and violence of a tornado, and the random pattern of destruction, often lead children to question, "Why me?" In one of the earliest studies of psychological impact, Bloch et al. (1956) studied children affected by a tornado that had destroyed a movie theater in Vicksburg, Mississippi, and found that one-third demon-strated significant psychological impairment. Factors mediating sever-ity of psychological distress were proximity to the theater, being injured, knowing somebody who was injured or killed, and parental psycholog-ical response.

Tornado Traumatic Reminders

Traumatic reminders of tornadoes include the annual publicity surround-ing the beginning of the tornado season, frequent announcements of tor-nado watches for the community, the periodic issuance of tornado warnings indicating actual formation of a tornado funnel, urgent guidance to take cover immediately, the ominous pulsation of the tornado siren, and the appearance of menacing cloud formations (especially when thick cloud banks take on a distinctive pea-green coloration). Other reminders are those that invoke memories of the brutality of a previous storm, such as thunder, lightning, and the crescendo of strong winds and torrential rains.

Wildfires

Wildfires may be ignited by random lightning strikes or careless flicks of burning embers; however, some wildfires are intentionally set as acts of arson. Wildfires can spread rampantly, especially when the ingredients of dry tinder and strong winds combine, thereby consuming large acreages of woodlands and wildlife. Wildfires are a growing natural hazard in most regions of the United States, posing a threat to life and property, particularly where native ecosystems meet developed areas. In populated areas, wildfires destroy homes, businesses, and schools. The secondary effects of a wildfire, including erosion, landslides, introduction of invasive species, and changes in water quality, are often more disastrous than the fire itself.

Preimpact Wildfire Stressors

Wildfires occur suddenly and unexpectedly. No formal warning systems exist. The path, speed, and damage potential of a wildfire are highly variable, depending on shifting wind patterns, rainfall, climate conditions, terrain, availability and density of dry fuel, human settlement patterns, and local firefighting capabilities and resources for combating wildfires.

Impact and Postimpact Wildfire Stressors

The swift and unrelenting approach of a firestorm, haphazardly changing directions or leaping across canyons and ridgelines, provokes fear and distress for those whose homes and neighborhoods are in harm's way. An encounter with fire and conflagration carries a particularly powerful threat of excruciating pain from burn injuries and horrific harm for self and loved ones. Communities may be called on to evacuate on short notice, forcing citizens to make urgent and agonizing decisions within minutes about where to go, when to leave, and what to take. McFarlane (1987), studying the effects of an Australian bush fire on 808 children, ages 5–12 years, found significant and sustained levels of psychological stress at 8 and 26 months after traumatic exposure.

Often, official warnings cannot keep pace with the dynamic and changeable nature of the wildfire threat. During the October 2007 San Diego wildfires, social media became an important source of warnings as the firestorms spread in many directions among residential areas perched on wooded ridges and hillsides. On May 5, 2011, the director of FEMA testified before Congress on the critical role of social media in disasters; the

San Diego wildfires contributed significantly to national recognition of the utility and timeliness of applying social media strategies to communicate risk and damage in real time during rapidly changing disaster events.

Wildfire Traumatic Reminders

The sound of crackling fire or the smell of smoke may trigger a sudden reliving and reexperiencing of a previous encounter with a wildfire. Other reminders may be those of the firefighting response, such as a wailing siren, the high-speed approach of a fire truck, the sound of low-flying aircraft, or media accounts of wildfires or house fires.

Pandemics

Infectious diseases, taken together, are a leading cause of death worldwide and remain a prominent cause of death in the United States and the developed world. Human existence has been punctuated by epidemics of infectious diseases that have shaped and transformed history. The Plague of Athens in the fifth century B.C. contributed to the defeat of the Athenians by Sparta in the Peloponnesian War. In the middle of the fourteenth century, one-third of the population in Europe died from the Black Death (bubonic plague). In the Americas, the rampant spread of smallpox, brought by explorers to the New World, paved the way for the European conquest of the indigenous peoples. The Spanish influenza pandemic of 1918–1919 killed between 50 and 100 million people worldwide, making it by far the deadliest disaster in human history. The pandemic of HIV/AIDS, first recognized in the 1980s, evolved to become the second leading cause of disability and the fourth leading cause of mortality worldwide by the end of the twentieth century.

For several years in the early 2000s, the predominant global infectious disease threat was believed to be the prospect of a pandemic H5N1 influenza, or avian flu. The first human case was diagnosed in 1997. The virus was associated with high lethality and complete absence of human immunity. No vaccine was available (Leavitt 2006). The H5N1 virus appeared capable of provoking an exaggerated immune response, with death occurring rapidly in persons across a wide age span, including many adolescents and young adults in robust health. One study revealed that the pathology of H5N1 influenza mimicked many of the salient characteristics of the 1918–1919 pandemic strain. However, as the infectious disease community was gearing up for H5N1 to become the next pandemic strain of influenza, in April 2009 the novel H1N1 virus was described; within several months, H1N1 became the dominant global strain of influenza. H5N1 has since vanished from media coverage (Turner et al. 2010).

The H1N1 pandemic in 2009 exhibited some unusual features, in that it was associated with major outbreaks in the northern hemisphere in the summer and autumn, and it caused widespread disease particularly among young people because of the lack of significant population immunity. Many of the hospitalizations and deaths were in those under age 60 years, and in a high proportion of cases of individuals who were hospitalized, the patients ended up in intensive care. Risk factors for infection, besides being young, were obesity, cardiovascular disease, and pregnancy. However, about one-third of those who died lacked any known risk factors (Turner et. al. 2010). The fortunate outcome was that the novel H1N1 turned out to be a relatively tame viral adversary — essentially equivalent in infectiousness and lethality to the previous seasonal flu strain that had been circulating since 1968. However, the global preparedness paid dividends in the rapid production of effective vaccines and the quick mounting of an effective public health response.

Preimpact Pandemic Stressors

Human behavior at the outbreak of a pandemic is a critical factor. Public education regarding pandemic disease should begin during early phases of the pandemic alert period. Once the pandemic is under way, warning periods will be reduced to days. The specific nature of the infectious agent, including its capability to infect (infectivity), cause clinical disease (pathogenicity), and kill its victims (virulence), will interplay with the population's ability to engage in preventive personal hygiene behaviors and to receive vaccines, antiviral medications, and medical treatments. The potential exists for global hardship, beginning even prior to the arrival of the pandemic, as citizens may begin to hoard food and essentials for the weeks of social distancing, thus creating acute shortages. Because the pandemic will sweep the globe, no areas will be spared. The inability to restock food and essential supplies may lead to widespread scarcity and possible outbreaks of violence. Lessons learned from H1N1 during the first 2 years of this new influenza strain will be invaluable for future encounters with a far deadlier pandemic strain (influenza strains undergo complete changeover about three times per century).

Impact and Postimpact Pandemic Stressors

Policy designed to prevent the spread of influenza must be implemented. Because person-to-person spread is the predominant mode of transmission of influenza virus, public health officials have suggested the employment of social distancing, with specific targeting of children and adolescents. This approach would require the closing of schools, an act that will represent a social stressor for children who are suddenly deprived of school-based peer relations and normal daily routines. If public health measures, including movement restrictions, are put into force, public reactions of anxiety, anger, and belligerence related to quarantine, social distancing, and perceived infringement on personal rights will likely proliferate.

Development of effective risk communications designed to educate the public regarding disease risks and preventive efforts may serve as a buffer against public fear and possible escalation to mass panic. Glass et al. (2006) reviewed public health strategies implemented during the 1957–1958 Asian flu pandemic and found that closing schools and keeping children at home reduced the "attack" rate by over 90%. School closure may be a critical and effective strategy to minimize contagion. During the advent of H1N1 in 2009, some school districts did indeed close schools for short periods of time.

When a pandemic moves through an area, uncertainty regarding possible exposure increases anxiety among families and their children. Individuals will be vulnerable to misinformation, contradictory data, and exaggerated news reports. If the media and public risk communications are not managed properly, the risk for chaos and the likelihood of a surge of fearful citizens on medical care facilities will be heightened. Individuals will be upset, demoralized, and likely to misattribute somatic symptoms to disease.

When the pandemic is at hand, large numbers of citizens will become ill, and many others will be tending to loved ones in the throes of disease. Some children and adolescents will directly witness the physical incapacitation and death of primary caretakers, family members, and close friends. The contagion of anxiety, fear, and overwhelming feelings of helplessness will extend across many family members as they struggle to access medical care and face an uncertain fate.

Pandemic Traumatic Reminders

Traumatic reminders of a pandemic include media stories about epidemic diseases, the annual arrival of the seasonal (nonpandemic) flu, rapid spread of other infectious diseases (familiar or newly emergent), and caring for a seriously ill relative or loved one.

The 2009 experience with the novel H1N1 provided a test of many public health, medical, and psychosocial strategies that were developed for a potentially highly virulent new strain of flu. Lessons learned must be carried forward because, despite the fortunate outcome in 2009, there will inevitably be a future encounter with a much more severe strain of influenza virus and the periodic introduction of newly emerging infectious diseases.

Nonintentional Human-Generated Disasters

The Centre for Research on the Epidemiology of Disasters (CRED) in Brussels, Belgium, hosts the international disaster database. Both natural disasters and nonintentional human-generated disasters are reported with a frequency of more than one per day. Most human-generated disasters involve a failure of technology, such as a collapse of a human construction (e.g., a building, tower, stadium, bridge, tunnel, or roadway); transportation accidents (e.g., air crashes, train or metro collisions, and bus accidents); industrial accidents (e.g., plant explosions, chemical leaks, and radiation releases). For the following subsections, we have selected diverse examples as illustrations of a structural collapse, a hazardous materials spill, and radiation releases.

Structural Failure: Bridge Collapse

During rush hour on August 1, 2007, the Interstate 35W bridge in Minneapolis, Minnesota, collapsed into the Mississippi River, breaking into five sections. Dozens of vehicles filled with commuters plunged into the wreckage or directly into the rapid current of the Mississippi River, resulting in 13 deaths and 145 injuries. The engineering firm URS Corporation was charged with negligence and in 2010 agreed to pay $52.4 million to settle claims from this purely human-generated event.

Hazardous Materials Spill

Following the explosion and incineration of British Petroleum's (BP's) Deepwater Horizon oil-drilling platform in the Gulf of Mexico in April 2010, the superstructure of the rig broke apart and sank to the sea bottom, severing the petroleum in-flow pipe. Millions of barrels of oil gushed unabated into the Gulf for a period of almost 100 days, polluting shorelines, fouling wildlife, and severely affecting coastal fishing and tourist industries. The extent of ecological damage to the Gulf of Mexico and the fragile coastal wetlands will take years to assess. BP's total payout for this human-generated disaster will likely reach $50 billion. BP paid $52 million to underwrite the psychosocial care of Gulf Coast residents and their families whose livelihoods were jeopardized by the spill.

Radiation Accidents

On April 26, 1986, a nuclear accident occurred at the Chernobyl nuclear power plant in the former Union of Soviet Socialist Republics (USSR) (now in the Ukraine, near the borders of Belarus and Russia), leading to a series of explosions and fires that destroyed the nuclear reactor and released a radioactive cloud, which spread quickly over Europe. Subsequently, several hundred thousand persons were uprooted from their homes and resettled outside the severely contaminated area (up to 30 kilometers). Radioactive fallout affected agriculture, forests, food products, plants, animal life, and waterways.

A dose-response relationship was evident; the greater the radiation exposure, the higher the rate of PTSD symptoms. Of the 150 plant workers, 28 emergency workers died from acute radiation and 20 others from probable radiation-related diseases (Baverstock and Williams 2006). An 18-year follow-up study of cleanup workers at the plant found that they had higher rates of depression, PTSD, and suicidal ideation compared with control subjects (Bromet et al. 2011). By 2005, an estimated 4,000 individuals exposed as children had developed thyroid cancer (Baverstock and Williams 2006). A study conducted in the city of Kiev compared 262 evacuees at age 19 who had been exposed as children to Chernobyl radiation with classmate and population-based controls. The exposed group was twice as likely to have an enlarged thyroid, cataracts, and major health problems (Bromet et al. 2009).

In March 2011, an extremely powerful earthquake just east of Japan sent a series of tsunami waves crashing onshore. The tsunami runup overtopped the seawalls protecting coastal nuclear reactors, damaging the cooling systems, which led to partial meltdown and radiation releases over populated areas. Among peacetime nuclear events, only the incineration of the nuclear reactor in Chernobyl created a greater human threat. Concerns were rekindled regarding the acute and chronic effects of a nuclear accident, especially in Japan, the nation that sustained the most severe consequences of radiation injury following bombing during World War II.

Young children are thought to be more vulnerable to radioactive exposure and subsequent cancer risk because of their high respiratory rate (Markenson and Reynolds 2006). The prolonged duration of psychological consequences following radiation accidents is notable, extending for more than 20 years in the case of the Chernobyl nuclear plant disaster (Beehler et al. 2008; Danzer and Weisshaar 2009; Greve et al. 2005; Havenaar et al. 1997).

Intentional Human-Generated Disasters

Terrorism

Types of Terrorism

Terrorism is the "unlawful use or threat of use of force or violence against individuals, property, governments, or societies, often to achieve political, religious, or ideological objectives" (U.S. Department of Defense 1990). Terrorists typically strike suddenly and unexpectedly, sometimes orchestrating simultaneous attacks on multiple targets, such as the 9/11 attacks on America, or a series of repeated events, such as suicide bombings in Israel or the 2002 sniper shootings in the Washington, D.C., area.

The increasing imbalance of power between the haves and the have-nots of the world has tempted those less technologically sophisticated to use acts of terror to redress the perceived imbalance. The armamentarium of weapons available to terrorists is increasing in variety, sophistication, lethality, accessibility, and ease of use. As the destructive potential of terrorist actions increases, so too does the likelihood that small groups of terrorists may achieve disproportionate power to overthrow rivals.

As the Institute of Medicine (2003) noted, "Terrorism is intended to provoke collective fear and uncertainty" (p. 27). This fear often spreads rapidly, like concentric circles from a rock thrown into a pond, affecting those directly impacted and extending out to other family members, the community at large, and sometimes the entire nation. Terrorist attacks, or even the threat of attack, may provoke severe psychological consequences associated with a perceived lack of control and an accompanying sense of helplessness. Terrorism has the capacity to erode the perception of community and national security; damage social solidarity and cohesion; and divide the community along racial, ethnic, economic, and religious fault lines.

Nuclear detonation. Detonation of a nuclear device is perhaps the most feared and anticipated terrorist act. The U.S. Department of Homeland Security has created a series of National Planning Scenarios, a comprehensive set of highly challenging disaster prototypes. The most destructive on the list is the detonation of a 10-kiloton nuclear device in a U.S. metropolitan area. If this scenario were to become a reality, the following would ensue: immediate and unprecedented physical destruction; widespread and life-threatening radioactive contamination; immediate death for tens of thousands of citizens due to initial blast injuries; and agonizing, protracted death over weeks to months among persons exposed to lethal doses of radiation. First responders would be exposed to high doses of radiation. Large numbers of persons would sustain painful but nonfatal blast injuries including burns, blistering, and possible blindness related to visual exposure. Radioactive contamination would occur because of either external exposure from the blast and fallout or internal exposure from ingestion of contaminated food and water. Depending on the device, the electromagnetic pulse could potentially disrupt or damage electronic databases, setting off a chain reaction of consequences for banking and critical infrastructure industries.

The psychological impact of a nuclear accident or explosion is related to the consequences of the blast and subsequent exposure of the population to radiation. As a consequence of radioactive exposure, enforced evacuation and relocation would be imperative, as large geographic expanses would be rendered uninhabitable in the aftermath of a nuclear detonation. These areas would experience destruction of the social fabric of the community, loss of infrastructure, and lifelong stigmatization. All facilities and services, including schools, businesses, and faith-based organizations, would cease to function. The concept of postdisaster restoration and reconstruction would be fundamentally altered by the inability of disaster survivors to repopulate their communities.

Chemical attack. The Department of Homeland Security has described a variety of potential scenarios around the theme of chemical attack. These include attacks using nerve agents, blister agents, toxic industrial chemicals, and chlorine gas. Historically, when chemical attacks and hazardous material spills have occurred, large numbers of persons in the vicinity have experienced fear regarding possible exposure. The hazardous agents are often colorless, odorless, and undetectable by human senses. The invisible nature of the threat creates uncertainty regarding the boundaries of exposure; many more persons seek screening than are actually at risk.

Chemical attacks typically involve release of aerosolized, heavier-than-air agents (e.g., sarin or chlorine) that accumulate close to the ground, creating greater risks for smaller children. Both due to their stature and their much greater surface-to-volume ratio, children are extremely susceptible to the health effects from a hazardous material release.

An additional stressor is the lack of information regarding risks and strategies for self-protection. Fear may provoke rapid, mass exodus from the area of perceived danger, leading to the possibility of injury as large numbers flee. When escape routes are perceived to be limited and entrapment is feared, the potential for mass panic is heightened. Large-scale surges on health care facilities may also occur. Depending on the nature of the chemical agent, a spectrum of physiological and psychological symptoms may become prominent, including skin lesions, respiratory distress, psychophysiological signs, and psychogenic symptoms. Concerns related to water and food contamination may add to fear reactions in the community.

On March 20, 1995, members of a doomsday cult released sarin gas, a neurotoxin, in the Tokyo subway system, killing 12 people. More than 5,500 persons, fearful of possible exposure, surged the health care system, rapidly overwhelming the medical resources. Psychological casualties outnumbered persons with actual sarin gas exposure, or with medical injuries sustained while rapidly evacuating the subway, by a ratio of almost 4:1 (Beaton et al. 2005). Many exposed individuals continued to manifest posttraumatic stress symptoms long after the event.

Explosives attack.   Conventional explosives attacks account for the vast majority of terrorist incidents. Improvised explosive devices (IEDs) have become a well-developed technology and highly effective means for causing both harm and horror. IEDs are small, mobile, and easily concealed, and they can be delivered with precision to the selected site of attack. Notable events that used conventional weapons and explosives include the 1995 Oklahoma City federal building bombings, the 1998 twin attacks on U.S. embassies in Kenya and Tanzania, the 2004 Madrid rail station bombing, and the 2008 Mumbai hotel invasion and occupation. Numerous conventional explosives attacks have occurred throughout the Middle East and inside Israel. The use of suicide bombers adds additional psychological dimensions (a human being willing to die for a cause) and provides the ultimate intelligent delivery system (the bomber selects the exact location for self-detonation to inflict the most grievous harm).

During the immediate impact period, the injuries and deaths caused by the blast wave, shrapnel and flying debris, and severe burns challenge the emergency response. Injured survivors may be trapped in collapsed structures or burning vehicles, or buried in rubble. To increase terror, secondary attacks may be timed to interfere with rescue efforts and to maim and kill first responders. Fears of recurrence lead to feelings of uncertainty and perceptions of imminent danger. Survivors and first responders are likely to be exposed to respiratory hazards from clouds of debris hovering over the impact zone and toxins that have been released into the atmosphere. The recovery, restoration, and reconstruction periods are prolonged. Survivors are at great psychological risk.

The Oklahoma City bombing graphically portrays the indiscriminate killing of innocents and the vulnerability of children. Of the 168 deaths, 19 were children. More than 200 children lost one or both parents. Over 60% of schoolchildren surveyed in nearby schools reported that they heard or felt the explosion, and more than one-third knew someone who was injured or killed (Pfefferbaum et al. 2002). Repeated television exposure to news reports of the bombing heightened the risk of post-traumatic stress symptoms (Pfefferbaum et al. 2001).

Bioterrorism. Bioterrorism has been defined as "the premeditated unlawful use or threat of use of a biological organism" with the intent to terrorize or to kill the defined enemy (Culpepper 2001). The Centers for Disease Control and Prevention (CDC) has identified the Category A bioterrorism agents of greatest concern: *Bacillus anthracis* (anthrax), *Yersinia pestis* (plague), *Francisella tularensis* (tularemia), smallpox virus, viral hemorrhagic fever viruses (e.g., Ebola and Marburg), and *Clostridium botulinum* (botulism) toxin (Culpepper 2001; Moran 2000a, 2000b). Scientists estimate that over 60 pathogens are capable of being weaponized with varying degrees of lethality and capacity for contagion. Depending on the infectious agent and its route of delivery to an unsuspecting community, a biological attack can result in a range of devastating effects (Shaw 2003; Shaw and Shaw 2004). If the infectious agent is transmissible from person to person, some of the outcomes may be analogous to those discussed earlier for pandemics.

Historically, the use of infectious agents as instruments of war was first noted at the time of the Black Death, in the mid-1300s, when a seaport town under siege attempted to repel the invaders by catapulting bodies infected with bubonic plague over the walls as bubonic germ warfare missiles (Cantor 2001). The first bioterrorist attack against the United States occurred in 1984 when a religious cult in Oregon contaminated the salad bars of 10 local restaurants with salmonella with the intention of incapacitating many residents so they would be unable to vote on a referendum unfavorable to the cult (Siegrist and Graham 1999). Although biological agents may be used to kill or severely sicken a population, they may also be used as a threat to extort a population to carry out the will of the biological terrorists.

Four methods may be used to deploy biological weapons: 1) food contamination, 2) water contamination, 3) aerosol delivery, and 4) person-to-person spread. Food and water supplies may also be contaminated through the poisoning of livestock (Stern 1999). Although many people assume that the technical expertise necessary to aerosolize microorganisms into dry powders or to create liquid slurries is beyond the capabilities of most terrorist groups, surface-modified anthrax spores were placed in envelopes and successfully mailed to U.S. media outlets and government officials in 2001, resulting in a total of five deaths among 22 persons who became infected. The CDC placed more than 35,000 postal workers, government employees, and media personnel on a prophylactic regimen of antibiotics. All three branches of the federal government were shut down for periods of time, and millions of pieces of mail were embargoed and delayed in processing. Tens of thousands of excess calls regarding potential hazardous materials were generated throughout the United States as citizens became excessively worried about white powders and puffy envelopes. Public anxiety was widespread, and large numbers of persons purchased and hoarded antibiotic medications.

Phases of Response to Terrorism

Preimpact terrorism stressors.   Acts of terrorism and bioterrorism occur sporadically and unpredictably, with very low prevalence in most areas. Terrorist acts are episodic, reflecting a manifestation of a political and ideological readiness to employ asymmetrical violence to achieve a group's goals. The predominant stressor for families and their children in the preimpact phase is uncertainty coupled with anxiety. An Israeli study noted that the uncertainty of where a terrorist act will occur results in comparable risks for posttraumatic stress symptoms for persons living in areas where terrorist attacks have and have not previously occurred (Shalev et al. 2006).

Impact phase terrorism stressors.   Each type of terrorist-perpetrated weapon of mass destruction is associated with a unique constellation of stressors. Understandably, survivors of terrorism experience extreme fear and distress compounded with intense feelings of helplessness, anger, and distrust. In the aftermath, survivors struggle to find meaning in the experience. Stressors include exposure to death on a mass scale (including deaths of children), personal harm, life-threatening illness, pain, and physical debility. Acts of terrorism separate and displace loved ones and disrupt the routines of everyday life, including school, home, and work. Feelings of biological fragility and psychological vulnerability are common.

Children are uniquely susceptible to human-generated acts of violence. Young children's diminutive size and limited motor skills hamper their ability to escape from harm's way during extreme events of all types. Children may not have the cognitive abilities to realistically evaluate risk; in fact, curiosity may actually attract them toward danger. The higher surface-to-volume ratio of children, compared with adults, increases a variety of risks, such as hypothermia, dehydration, and exposure to hazardous materials.

Postimpact terrorism stressors. The degree of devastation resulting from terrorist attacks ranges from highly focused damage from an IED to the wholesale destruction of a community following a nuclear detonation, bioterrorism, or a chemical attack. Depending on the scope and extent of the devastation rendered by a terrorist act, the community will confront a fairly predictable litany of secondary stressors (Shaw 2003; Shaw and Shaw 2004). Families and communities should not underestimate the cumulative effects of terror, fear, and uncertainty precipitated by terrorist actions. Subsequent to a major terrorist attack are the issues related to evacuation, displacement, relocation, and rebuilding. Communities may experience loss of access to basic needs such as food and water, and disruption of vital services such as electrical power, transportation, and health care. Efforts to contend with these adversities may deplete a community's resilience, coping, and emotional resources. In the aftermath, many families may grapple with untimely or gruesome death, disabling illness or injury, or loss of home or valued possessions. Family functioning may change, as manifested by marital problems, domestic violence, substance abuse, financial hardship, and demoralization. Multiple, compounding losses are common following human-generated disasters, frequently leading to feelings of depression and vulnerability. Rates of substance abuse, delinquent acts, and interpersonal violence may rise.

In the aftermath of terrorism, ecological and psychosocial disruption will continue unabated long after the impact phase. Family support and social networks may disintegrate as people are displaced and relocated. Survivors may be relegated to living in public shelters, with great uncertainty regarding their ability to return to home, school, or work. Life and family routines will be dismantled. Perceived personal and family security will be undermined.

Terrorism Traumatic Reminders

Individuals who have directly experienced terrorist attacks are vulnerable to sudden, unexpected exposure to traumatic reminders that resonate with the trauma event.

War-Related Trauma

The most powerful human-generated disaster is war. War is one of the constants of human history, a product of the competitive struggle for territory, resources, and power (Durant and Durant 1968). At any time in history, war is an ongoing reality for some populations and a seemingly remote possibility for others. War may come suddenly and unexpectedly to populations not previously engaged in conflict. War invariably shreds the socioeconomic fabric of the community, disrupting moral codes, embedded patterns of relationships, and shared values (de Jong 2002). The impact of war cuts across all levels of society. Individuals exposed to war-related traumas experience the same range of psychological responses as those exposed to other forms of trauma.

As civil wars have proliferated, civilians have become the main casualties. According to estimates in 2009, more than 1 billion children lived in countries affected by armed conflict, equivalent to one-seventh of the world's population (UNICEF 2009). Since 1990, conflicts have killed 3.6 million people, and 45% of these have been children. Hundreds of thousands of children are caught up in armed conflict. Some children are conscripted to serve as soldiers. Others are displaced by war, becoming refugees or internally displaced persons (IDPs). Children in war-torn countries suffer sexual violence, abuse, and exploitation.

Children may be maimed or killed by the explosive remnants of war. UNICEF estimates that 90% of global conflict-related deaths since 1990 have been noncombatant civilians. Women and children comprise 80% of civilian war-related deaths (UNICEF 2005). An estimated 2 million children have been killed in wars, 5 million have been disabled, and 12 million have been left homeless (UNICEF 1997). Children may also suffer from exposure to genocidal behavior. A national survey of 1,547 Rwandans ages 8–19 years revealed that 90% had witnessed killing, 30% had witnessed sexual assaults, 35% had lost a family member, and 15% had hidden under a corpse to protect themselves (Neugebauer et al. 2009). The authors estimated that 54%–62% of the survey participants had probable PTSD. As with other types of disasters, the risk of PTSD was directly related to level of exposure to armed conflict and its

TABLE 2–2.   **Stressors faced by children in wartime**

Lack of adequate food, shelter, and medical care

Separation from caregivers, family, and loved ones

Exposure to violence and brutal deaths

Injury to self

Injury or death of a family member

Forced displacement from home

Loss of community, school, and social supports

Exploitation

Physical or sexual abuse

Source.   Duncan and Arntson 2004.

consequences. The risk for PTSD approaches 100% for children with the highest level of exposure.

War-related traumas are diverse, accumulate over time, and have an immediate and enduring psychological effect on children. The most powerful predictors of adverse psychological effects of war are the intensity and the duration of exposure to war-related traumatic events (Hadi and Llabre 1998; Neugebauer et al. 2009; Thabet and Vostanis 1999; Vizek-Vidovic et al. 2000). Estimates of the prevalence of posttraumatic stress symptomatology among children exposed to war-related stressors vary broadly, from 10% to 90%, including nonspecific anxiety disorders, PTSD, depression, disruptive behaviors, and somatic symptoms (De Jong 2002; Goldstein et al. 1997; Hadi and Llabre 1998). In war, however, children more often die from starvation, sickness, and the stress of flight than from physical injury and violence. Thus, some evidence suggests that efforts need to focus on reducing exposure to both war-related trauma and the secondary stressors of war (i.e., graphic media coverage, loss of food and shelter, economic uncertainty, and the lack of appropriate medical and pediatric support services). Stressors faced by children in wartime are noted in Table 2–2.

Refugees and Internally Displaced Persons

Approximately 80%–90% of all victims of warfare today are women and children (UNICEF 2009). Many seek safety and shelter to escape from war, homelessness, hunger, disease, and persecution. An estimated 20 million children have been displaced by armed conflict either as refugees or as IDPs (UNICEF 2009). Civilians are defined as refugees when they cross an international frontier to seek sanctuary in another country. For example, 75,000 Bosnian refugees, one-third of whom were children, sought asylum in Sweden (Goldin et al. 2001). The exile experience for these refugees was marked by stages: living in temporary sorting camps, followed by transfer to crowded military barracks. Refugees in flight are frequently exposed to brutal death, the traumatic effects of perilous flight, interpersonal violence, physical injury, mutilation, rape, and malnutrition. While fleeing danger and seeking refuge, children may become separated from their families, placing them in danger of exposure to violence, malnutrition, disease, forced recruitment, human trafficking, child labor, sexual exploitation, and death. In addition to culture shock, refugees face loss of native language and customs, xenophobia, poverty, and downward social and professional mobility.

Many refugees are temporarily settled in camp environments, where they normally receive food, shelter, and a place of safety from the host country. Conditions in the camps, however, are such that individuals experience crowding, poor nutrition, poverty, enforced passivity, unemployment, boredom, discrimination, and continuous exposure to violence and death as parts of the daily landscape. The refugees often lack a formal legal identity, a factor that makes them attractive to human traffickers. The United Nations and other humanitarian organizations work to help refugees restart their lives in a new place or eventually return home. Studies have revealed that war refugee children and their families have a range of psychiatric disorders, including PTSD, mood disorders, anxiety reactions, disruptive behaviors, and somatoform disorders (Goldin et al. 2001; Weine et al. 1995).

More than 31 million women and children have been classified as IDPs (UNICEF 2009). IDPs take flight from home communities but seek shelter and safety elsewhere within the geopolitical boundaries of their own country. Because they do not traverse an international border, IDPs are not afforded some of the protections offered to refugees. Instead, IDPs have minimal legal or physical protection and a very uncertain future, existing as outcasts within their own countries. IDPs are trapped in ongoing internal conflict. The domestic government, which may view the uprooted people as enemies of the state, retains ultimate power over their fate. No specific international legal instruments cover human rights for IDPs. General agreements such as the Geneva Conventions are difficult to apply and virtually impossible to enforce. International supervision of IDP health status is not available, and humanitarian agencies may be barred from providing support. Moreover, philanthropic donors are frequently reluctant to intervene in internal

TABLE 2–3. **Top 10 countries for refugees and internally displaced persons (IDPs)**

Refugees, 2008			IDPs, 2009		
Rank	Country	Number	Rank	Country	Number
1	Pakistan	1,780,935	1	Sudan	4,900,000
2	Syria	1,105,698	2	Colombia	3,300,000–4,900,000
3	Iran	980,109	3	Iraq	2,760,000
4	Germany	582,735	4	Democratic Republic of Congo	1,900,000
5	Jordan	500,413	5	Somalia	1,500,000
6	Chad	330,510	6	Pakistan	1,200,000
7	Tanzania	321,909	7	Turkey	954,000–1,201,000
8	Kenya	320,605	8	Zimbabwe	570,000–1,000,000
9	China	300,967	9	India	500,000
10	United Kingdom	292,097	10	Myanmar	470,000

Source. UNICEF 2009.

conflicts or offer sustained assistance. The top 10 countries with refugees and the top 10 countries with IDPs are listed in Table 2–3, and trauma risk factors for children in these groups are noted in Table 2–4.

Child Soldiers

Of particular interest to mental health professionals who work with child survivors of trauma are child soldiers. Child soldiers are both victims of war and perpetrators of violence. More than 300,000 child soldiers younger than 18 years are engaged in various conflicts in more than 50 countries (Office of the Special Representative of the Secretary-General for Children and Armed Conflict 2005). Estimates suggest that Africa alone has 100,000 child soldiers, who have participated in warring conflicts in Sierra Leone, Liberia, Mozambique, Somalia, Congo,

---

TABLE 2–4.   Trauma risks for refugee and internally displaced children

---

Risk of malnutrition

Increased risk of disease and physical injury

Lack of protection and increased risk of physical or sexual violence

Discrimination

Lack of educational opportunities

Emotional risks due to exposure to death, injury, multiple losses, bereavement, loss of community and/or country affiliation

Special situations with higher risks for refugee and internally displaced children

    Coercion to become a child soldier

    Child labor (hard physical labor, duties involving high danger, begging, prostitution)

    Slavery following sale by child traffickers

Source.   United Nations High Commissioner for Refugees 2006.

and Uganda. The use of children for military purposes has precedents in ancient history. Well-known historical examples include David's service to King Saul, French drummer boys in Napoleon's army, young boys who served as so-called powder monkeys on the ships of the British Royal Navy, and the Hitler Youth (Hitler-Jugend) in Nazi Germany who were formed into combat units for the defense of Berlin.

Children are especially vulnerable to recruitment because of their emotional and physical immaturity. Many children are refugees, or they are displaced from home, separated from families, or orphaned. These children have little means of support or access to education or employment. Children may be abducted or seized from the streets, villages, schools, and orphanages. The child militias become a source of security, a surrogate family, and a guarantor of meals, clothing, and shelter. Once recruited, children often serve as porters, cooks, couriers, spotters, spies, human shields, and even suicide bombers. Technological advances in weaponry have led to the development of lightweight automatic weapons that are simple to operate and can easily be used by children. In battle, child soldiers are often pushed forward as cannon fodder and suffer high casualty rates from enemy fire and land mines.

Many child soldiers have been forced to commit acts of violence to prove their fidelity to the group. Exposure to brutal aggressive violence against others at such an early age may damage and derange their moral sense regarding violence (de Silva and Hobbs 2001; Shaw and Harris 1994). The child warriors are often the most feared of all soldiers because they have been acculturated to violence and have few scruples about killing (Shaw and Harris 2003a, 2003b). The derivative effects of exposure to war-related stressors on the developing child are far ranging and may affect the elaboration and consolidation of personality traits, identity formation, adaptive and coping mechanisms, internalized standards of right and wrong, intrinsic mechanisms for modulating aggressive impulses, and the child's habitual mode of relating to others. This exposure also has enduring neurobiological consequences.

Bayer et al. (2007) studied 169 former Ugandan and Congolese child soldiers. The average child soldier had been violently abducted into the Lord's Resistance Army at 12 years of age and had served, on average, for 3 years. Three-fourths of these children reported one or more of these experiences: threats of being killed, serious injury, or witnessing a friend or family member being killed. Over half had killed others. The authors noted that child soldiers with the most posttraumatic stress symptoms were less likely to be open to reconciliation with the enemy and harbored more aggressive vengeful fantasies. The authors concluded that posttraumatic stress might prevent these children from being able to deal with and overcome feelings of hatred and revenge and thus lessen the opportunity to seek peaceful ways to resolve conflict.

Betancourt et al. (2010) followed 156 child soldiers from Sierra Leone (ages 10–18; 12% female) over a 2-year period in an effort to delineate their level of psychosocial adjustment and to identify risk and protective factors. Nearly all of the children (99%) had been conscripted and had an average length of service of 5 years. The degree of hostility in the youth was correlated with exposure to war-related violence, being wounded, having killed someone, and being a victim of rape. Family and community acceptance and school retention were correlated with prosocial attitudes.

Growing evidence indicates that some child soldiers are quite resilient. Klasen et al. (2010) studied 330 former Ugandan child soldiers (ages 11–17; 48.5% female) who had served in militias for an average of 20 months (and had been away from their armed militias for an average of 32 months). Thirty percent did not meet criteria for PTSD and depression, and did not manifest clinically significant behavioral and emotional problems. The posttraumatic resilience was thought to be mediated by multiple factors, including reduced exposure to domestic and community violence, decreased revenge motivation, decreased peritraumatic dissociation, decreased self-attributions of guilt, improved socioeconomic circumstances, and more perceived spiritual support.

Currently, human rights advocates and international support groups are encouraging the adoption of the 1998 Rome Statute of the International Criminal Court, which makes it a war crime to conscript or enlist children younger than 15 years of age for armed conflict. However, adoption of this international legislation will not ensure an end to recruitment. The campaign against the exploitation of children as combatants must also include processes for sensitively reintegrating former child combatants into civil society. Government and international resources must focus on developing programs to ensure the provision of psychosocial and medical care, educational opportunities, literacy, and occupational skills training for former child soldiers. These reintegration components, however, have received less financial support than disarmament and demobilization efforts, an imbalance that can lead to further violence (UNICEF 2005).

■ Key Clinical Points

- ■ Disaster is a severe ecological and psychosocial disruption that greatly exceeds the coping capacity of the altered community.

- ■ Disasters are generally divided into two broad categories: natural disasters and human-generated disasters.

- ■ Human-generated disasters are subdivided into those that are nonintentional (technological failures and "accidents") and those that are intentional (acts of terrorism, armed conflict, and war).

- ■ A multidimensional disaster occurs when elements of a natural disaster (an act of nature) and a nonintentional human-generated disaster combine and co-occur.

- ■ Disaster impact is related to the scale and scope of the event.

- ■ The disaster life cycle consists of preimpact, impact, and postimpact phases.

- ■ Each type of disaster can be described in terms of a unique constellation of preimpact, impact, and postimpact phase stressors and trauma reminders.

References

Ahearn FL, Cohen RE: Disasters and Mental Health: An Annotated Bibliography (DHHS Publ No ADM 84-1311). Rockville, MD, Center for Mental Health Services, 1985

Basoglu M, Kilic C, Salcioglu E, et al: Prevalence of posttraumatic stress disorder and comorbid depression in earthquake survivors in Turkey: an epidemiological study. J Trauma Stress 17:133–144, 2004

Basoglu M, Salcioglu E, Livanou M: Advances in Our Understanding of Earthquake Trauma and Its Treatment: A Self-Help Model of Mental Health Care for Survivors, in Mental Health and Disasters. Edited by Neria Y, Galea S, Norris FH. Cambridge, UK, Cambridge University Press, 2009, pp 396–418

Baverstock K, Williams D: The Chernobyl accident 20 years on: an assessment of the health consequences and the international response. Environ Health Perspect 114:1312–1317, 2006

Bayer CP, Klasen F, Adam H: Association of trauma and PTSD symptoms with openness to reconciliation and feelings of revenge among former Ugandan and Congolese child soldiers. JAMA 298:555–559, 2007

Beaton R, Stergachis A, Oberle M, et al: The sarin gas attacks on the Tokyo subway: 10 years later/lesson learned. Traumatology 11:103–119, 2005

Becker-Blease KA, Turner HA, Finkelhor D: Disasters, victimization, and children's mental health. Child Dev 81:1040–1053, 2010

Beehler GP, Baker JA, Falkner K, et al: A multilevel analysis of long-term psychological distress among Belarusians affected by the Chernobyl disaster. Public Health 122:1239–1249, 2008

Betancourt TS, Borisova II, Williams TP, et al: Sierra Leone's former child soldiers: a follow-up study of psychosocial adjustment and community reintegration. Child Dev 81:1077–1095, 2010

Bloch DA, Perry SE, Silber E: Some factors in the emotional reactions of children to disaster. Am J Psychiatry 113:416–422, 1956

Breslau N, Kessler RC, Chilcoat HD, et al: Trauma and posttraumatic stress disorder in the community: the 1996 Detroit Area Survey of Trauma. Arch Gen Psychiatry 55:626–632, 1998

Bromet EJ, Taormina DP, Guey LT, et al: Subjective health legacy of the Chornobyl accident: a comparative study of 19-year olds in Kyiv. BMC Public Health 9:417, 2009

Bromet EJ, Havenaar JM, Guey LT: A 25 year retrospective review of the psychological consequences of the Chernobyl accident. Clin Oncol 23:297–305, 2011

Cantor NF: In the Wake of the Plague. New York, Free Press, 2001

Cohen JA, Jaycox LH, Walker DW, et al: Treating traumatized children after Hurricane Katrina: Project Fleur-de lis. Clin Child Fam Psychol Rev 12:55–64, 2009

Copeland WE, Keeler G, Angold A, et al: Traumatic events and posttraumatic stress in childhood. Arch Gen Psychiatry 64:577–584, 2007

Cordasco KM, Eisenman DP, Glik DC, et al: They blew the levee: distrust of authorities among Hurricane Katrina evacuees. J Health Care Poor Underserved 18:277–282, 2007

Costello ED, Messer SC, Bird HR, et al: The prevalence of serious emotional disturbance: a re-analysis of community studies. J Child Fam Stud 7:411–431, 1998

Culpepper RC: Agents of bioterrorism, in Planning for Bioterrorism: Behaviors and Mental Health Response to Weapons of Mass Destruction and Mass Disruption. Bethesda, MD, Center for the Study of Traumatic Stress, Department of Psychiatry, Uniformed Services University of the Health Sciences, 2001, pp 17–34

Danzer AM, Weisshaar N: The long run consequences of the Chernobyl catastrophe on subjective well-being and mental health in Ukraine: evidence from two large data sets. Working paper presented at the Annual Conference of the European Association of Labour Economists, Tallinn, Estonia, 2009

De Jong J: Trauma, War and Violence: Public Mental Health in Socio-Cultural Context. New York, Kluver Academic/Plenum, 2002

de Silva DGH, Hobbs CJ: Conscription of children in armed conflict. BMJ 322:1372, 2001

Durant W, Durant A: The Lessons of History. New York, Simon & Schuster, 1968

Erikson K: Disaster at Buffalo Creek: loss of communality at Buffalo Creek. Am J Psychiatry 133:302–305, 1976

Giannopoulou I, Strouthos M, Smith P, et al: Post-traumatic stress reactions of children and adolescents exposed to the Athens 1999 earthquake. Eur Psychiatry 21:160–166, 2006

Glass RJ, Glass LM, Beyeler WE, et al: Targeted social distancing design for pandemic influenza. Emerg Infect Dis 12:1671–1681, 2006

Glickman TS (ed): Glossary of Meteorology. Boston, MA, American Meteorological Society, 2000

Goldin S, Lein L, Persson LA, et al: Stories of prewar, war and exile: Bosnian refugee children in Sweden. Med Confl Surviv 17:25–47, 2001

Goldstein RD, Wampler NS, Wise PH: War experience and distress symptoms of Bosnian children. Pediatrics 100:873–878, 1997

Greve KW, Bianchini KJ, Doane BM, et al: Psychological evaluation of the emotional effects of a community toxic exposure. J Occup Environ Med 47:51–59, 2005

Hadi FA, Llabre MM: The Gulf crisis experience of Kuwaiti children: psychological and cognitive factors. J Trauma Stress 11:45–56, 1998

Havenaar JM, Rumyantzeva GM, Van den Brink W, et al: Long-term mental health effects of the Chernobyl disaster: an epidemiologic survey in two former Soviet regions. Am J Psychiatry 154:1605–1607, 1997

Institute of Medicine: Preparing for the Psychological Consequences of Terrorism: A Public Health Strategy. Washington, DC, National Academies Press, 2003

Kessler RC, Sonnega A, Bromet E, et al: Posttraumatic stress disorder in the National Comorbidity Survey. Arch Gen Psychiatry 52:1048–1060, 1995

Kessler RC, Galea S, Jones RT, et al: Mental illness and suicidality after Hurricane Katrina. Bull World Health Organ 84:930–939, 2006

Kilmer RP, Gil-Rivas V: Responding to the needs of children and families after a disaster: linkages between unmet needs and caregiver functioning. Am J Orthopsychiatry 80:135–142, 2010

Klasen F, Oettingen G, Daniels J, et al: Posttraumatic resilience in former Ugandan child soldiers. Child Dev 81:1096–1113, 2010

Klotzbach PJ, Gray WM: Extended range forecast of Atlantic seasonal hurricane activity and U.S. landfall strike probability for 2006. 2005. Fort Collins, Colorado State University. Available at: http://hurricane.atmos.colostate.edu/Forecasts/2006. Accessed August 18, 2011.

Kuwabara H, Shioiri T, Toyabe SI, et al: Factors impacting on psychological distress and recovery after the 2004 Niigata-Chuetsu earthquake, Japan: community-based study. Psychiatry Clin Neurosci 62:503–507, 2008

Lau JTF, Yu X, Zhang J, et al: Psychological distress among adolescents in Chengdu, Sichuan at 1 month after the 2008 Sichuan earthquake. J Urban Health 87:504–523, 2010

Lay T, Kanamori H, Ammon CJ, et al: The great Sumatra-Andaman earthquake of 26 December 2004. Science 308:1127–1133, 2005

Leavitt MO: Pandemic planning update: a report from Secretary Michael O. Leavitt. Washington, DC, Department of Health and Human Services, March 13, 2006

Markenson D, Reynolds S: American Academy of Pediatrics Committee on Pediatric Emergency Medicine; Task Force on Terrorism: The pediatrician and disaster preparedness. Pediatrics 117: e340–e362, 2006

McFarlane AC: Posttraumatic phenomena in a longitudinal study of children following a natural disaster. J Am Acad Child Adolesc Psychiatry 26:764–769, 1987

McLaughlin KA, Fairbank JA, Gruber MJ, et al: Serious emotional disturbance among youths exposed to Hurricane Katrina 2 years postdisaster. J Am Acad Child Adolesc Psychiatry 48:1069–1078, 2009

Moran GJ: Biological terrorism: are we prepared? Part I. Emergency Medicine 2:14–38, 2000a

Moran GJ: Biological terrorism: are we prepared? Part II. Emergency Medicine 3:110–115, 2000b

National Hurricane Center: Hurricane preparedness: watches and warnings. Available at: http://www.nhc.noaa.gov/HAW2/english/forecast/warnings.shtml. Accessed November 15, 2011.

Neugebauer R, Fisher PW, Turner JB, et al: Posttraumatic stress reactions among Rwanda children and adolescents in the early aftermath of genocide. Int J Epidemiol 38:1033–1045, 2009

Norris FH, Wind LH: The experience of disaster: trauma, loss, adversities, and community effects, in Mental Health and Disasters. Edited by Neria Y, Galea S, Norris FH. Cambridge, UK, Cambridge University Press, 2009, pp 29–44

Office of the Special Representative of the Secretary-General for Children and Armed Conflict: Protection of children affected by armed conflict. Report to the General Assembly A/60/335. New York, United Nations, 2005

Pfefferbaum B, Nixon SJ, Tivis RD, et al: Television exposure in children after a terrorist incident. Psychiatry 64:202–211, 2001

Pfefferbaum B, Doughty DE, Reddy C, et al: Exposure and peritraumatic response as predictors of posttraumatic stress in children following the 1995 Oklahoma City bombing. J Urban Health 79:354–363, 2002

Pynoos RS, Goenjian AK, Steinberg AM: A public mental health approach to the post disaster treatment of children and adolescents. Child Adolesc Psychiatr Clin N Am 7:195–210, 1998

Quarantelli EL: Catastrophes Are Different From Disasters: Some Implications for Crisis Planning and Managing Drawn From Katrina. 2006. Available at: http://understandingkatrina.ssrc.org/Quarantelli. Accessed August 18, 2011.

Schoenbaum M, Butler B, Kataoka S, et al: Promoting mental health recovery after Hurricanes Katrina and Rita: what can be done at what cost. Arch Gen Psychiatry 66:906–914, 2009

Shalev AY, Tuval R, Frenkiel-Fishman et al: Psychological responses to continuous terror: a study of two communities in Israel. Am J Psychiatry 163:667–673, 2006

Shaw JA: Children exposed to war/terrorism. Clinical Child and Family Psychology Review 6(4):237–246, 2003

Shaw JA, Harris JJ: Children of war and children at war: child victims of terrorism in Mozambique, in Trauma and Disaster. Edited by Ursano RJ, McCaughey BE, Fullerton CS. London, Cambridge University Press, 1994, pp 287–305

Shaw JA, Harris J: Children exposed to war/terrorism. Clin Child Fam Psychol Rev 6:237–246, 2003a

Shaw J, Harris J: Children of war and children at war: child victims of terror in Mozambique, in Terrorism and Disaster. Edited by Ursano RJ, Fullerton CS, Norwood A. Cambridge, UK, Cambridge University Press, 2003b, pp 41–57

Shaw JA, Shaw S: The psychological effects of a community-wide disaster on children: planning for bioterrorism, in Bioterrorism: Psychological and Public Health Interventions. Edited by Ursano R. London, Cambridge University Press, 2004, pp 144–164

Shaw JA, Applegate B, Tanner S, et al: Psychological effects of Hurricane Andrew on an elementary school population. J Am Acad Child Adolesc Psychiatry 34:1185–1192, 1995

Shaw JA, Applegate B, Schorr C: Twenty-one-month follow-up study of school-age children exposed to Hurricane Andrew. J Am Acad Child Adolesc Psychiatry 35:359–364, 1996

Shaw JA, Espinel Z, Shultz JM: Children: Stress, Trauma and Disasters. Tampa, FL, Disaster Life Support Publishing, 2007

Shultz JM, Espinel Z, Flynn BW, et al: Deep Prep: All-Hazards Disaster Behavioral Health Training. Tampa, FL, Disaster Life Support Publishing, 2007

Siegrist DM, Graham JM (eds): Countering Biological Terrorism in the U.S.: An Understanding of Issues and Status. Dobbs Ferry, NY, Oceana Publications, 1999

Stern J: The prospect of domestic bioterrorism. Emerg Infect Dis 5:517–522, 1999

Sumer N, Karanci AN, Berument SK, et al: Personal resources, coping self-efficacy, and quake exposure as predictors of psychological distress following the 1999 earthquake in Turkey. J Trauma Stress 18:331–342, 2005

Thabet AA, Vostanis P: Post-traumatic stress reactions in children of war. J Child Psychol Psychiatry 40:385–391, 1999

Toole MJ: Mass population displacement: a global public health challenge. Infect Dis Clin North Am 9:353–366, 1990

Turner SJ, Doherty PC, Kelso A: Q&A: H1N1 pandemic influenza: what's new? BMC Biol 8:130, 2010

UNICEF: The State of the World's Children 1997. New York, UNICEF, 1997. Available at: www. unicef.org/sowc97. Accessed August 16, 2011.

UNICEF: The State of the World's Children 2005: Children Under Threat. New York, UNICEF, 2005

UNICEF: Machel Study 10-Year Strategic Review: Children and Conflict in a Changing World. New York, UNICEF, 2009

United Nations Development Program: Reducing Disaster Risk: A Challenge for Development. New York, John S Swift, 2004

United Nations High Commissioner for Refugees: Measuring Protection by Numbers 2005. Geneva, United Nations High Commissioner for Refugees, November 2006. Available at: www.unhcr.org/basic/BASICS3bo28097c. html.

Ursano RJ, Fullerton CS, Benedek DM: What is psychopathology after disasters? Considerations about the nature of the psychological and behavioral consequences of disasters, in Mental Health and Disasters. Edited by Neria Y, Galea S, Norris FH. Cambridge, UK, Cambridge University Press, 2009, pp 131–142

U.S. Department of Defense: Military Operations in Low Intensity Conflict (Field Manual 100-20/Air Force Pamphlet 3-20). Departments of the Army and Air Force, December 5, 1990

Vizek-Vidovic V, Kuterovac-Jagodic G, Arambasic L: Posttraumatic symptomatology in children exposed to war. Scand J Psychol 41:297–306, 2000

Weine S, Becker DF, McGlashan TH, et al: Adolescent survivors of ethnic cleansing, observations on the first year in America. J Am Acad Child Adolesc Psychiatry 34:1153–1159, 1995

Wickrama KA, Kaspar V: Family context of mental health risk in tsunami-exposed adolescents: findings from a pilot study in Sri Lanka. Soc Sci Med 64:713–723, 2007

World Health Organization, Division of Mental Health: Psychosocial Consequences of Disaster: Prevention and Management. Geneva, World Health Organization, 1992

Zunin LM, Myers D: Training Manual for Human Service Workers in Major Disasters, 2nd Edition (DHHS Publ No ADM 90-538). Washington, DC, Department of Health and Human Services, Substance Abuse and Mental Health Services Administration, Center for Mental Health Services, 2000

The Context of Trauma

■ Recognize that psychological effects of trauma are mediated through a myriad of contextual factors.

■ Describe the major components of the disaster ecology model.

■ Recognize the relationship between level of exposure to disaster and severity of psychological consequences.

■ Identify the individual factors that mediate the child's response to the traumatizing effect of disaster.

■ Identify the family factors that mediate the child's response to the traumatizing effect of disaster.

■ Identify the role of community and societal factors mediating the child's response to the traumatizing effect of disaster.

Introduction

The child's psychological response to a potentially injurious or life-threatening disaster is influenced by a complex variety of contextual factors operating at individual, family, community, and societal levels. Within each level, risk factors exacerbate psychological responses, while protective factors mitigate the impact of disaster.

For children, individual factors include age, gender, medical and psychiatric history, previous history of trauma, and level of functioning before and during the disaster. The child filters the disaster experience differently depending on his or her current stage of cognitive development and level of understanding of disaster causation.

Family factors are particularly relevant determinants of the child's response to trauma and disaster. The factors include family structure

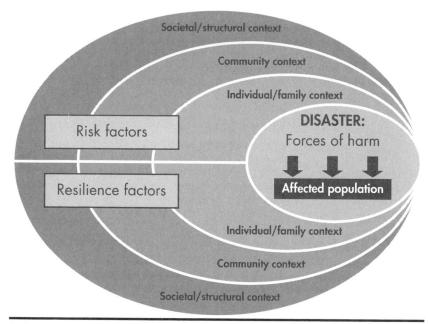

FIGURE 3–1.   Disaster ecology model.

Source.   Shaw JA, Espinel Z, Shultz JM: *Children: Stress, Trauma and Disasters.* Tampa, FL, Disaster Life Support Publishing, 2007.

and family cohesiveness, communication patterns, parental response to disaster impact, and postdisaster family functioning. Community and societal factors include social support networks, culture, ethnicity, socioeconomic status, political structure and governance, and postdisaster community functioning.

Disaster Ecology Model

Disaster ecology incorporates the principles of social ecology and examines the interrelationships and interdependence of the social, psychological, anthropological, cultural, geographic, and economic consequences of disasters and extreme events (Shultz et al. 2007).

Many elements of the environment exert influences on a child's life and behavior. Children exist within a family unit that connects to other systems: extended family, friends and peers, local neighborhoods, schools, and the encompassing community. The strongest influences tend to come from those life systems that are closest to the child. For many children, the family unit is the most central, followed by the peer network and then by

TABLE 3–1. Disaster ecology model: major components

Component	Description
Forces of harm	Disaster hazards
Human population[a] in harm's way	Children and families directly threatened or impacted by the forces of harm, or indirectly sustaining loss and change associated with the disaster event
Ecological context	Risk and resilience factors, operating at many levels, that influence the degree of physical and psychological harm sustained during a disaster or extreme event

[a]Primary focus for the purposes of this book is on children and families.

the school community and local neighborhood. The social ecological perspective supports the contention that the child's response to disaster and traumatic experience is shaped by the complex matrix of risk and protective factors comprising the ecological context. The disaster ecology model is depicted in Figure 3–1, and the major components of the model are noted in Table 3–1.

Disaster Exposure

For children, disaster exposure is a product of their direct encounter with the forces of harm and their geographic proximity to the epicenter of impact. Children may sustain personal injury during the impact or rescue phase. Some children will experience desperate anguish when separated from caregivers, whether briefly or for a protracted period of time. Some will lose a loved one, possibly a parent, in the disaster. Children may witness injury to family members at close range or observe grotesque, incongruous scenes in their home neighborhoods. When disaster is close at hand, many children will have intense fear reactions, at times rising to the level of panic sensations. Some children may perceive life threat, believing they are going to die or be horrifically hurt. Children's attention will also be riveted on the behaviors and emotional responses of their parents and the important adults in their lives; they will look to these powerful figures for reassurance and cues for how to act; frequently, children reproduce the same reactions they observe. Taken together, these various elements represent a constellation of evidence-based risk factors for psychological distress and impairment for children exposed to disaster. Factors that shape the psychosocial responses to disaster are listed in Table 3–2.

Individuals most exposed to disaster in terms of proximity, dose, and duration of exposure are the most likely to be affected and experience psychological morbidity. Exposure and psychological distress, however, extend far beyond the impact zone to affect persons distant from the scene and remotely connected to the event.

The persons who experience psychological reactions may be numerous, and the affected persons are remarkably diverse. For the child, the intensity of psychological impact relates not only to the extent of direct exposure sustained by his or her family, but also to the degree of social connectedness with the direct impact victims. The closer the interpersonal bonds are, the greater the psychological consequences for the individual.

For some disasters, gradations of exposure can be defined objectively — for example, geographic distance from the eye of a land-falling hurricane, or the epicenter of an earthquake, or the precise point of explosion of a terrorist bomb. Other dimensions of exposure are more subjective, such as social relatedness to disaster survivors or the role played by disaster responders. Regardless, gradations of disaster exposure create a hierarchy of stress and trauma.

Generally, the most intense exposure and the highest likelihood for psychological morbidity are found for children and families who are severely injured or who lose a close family member or friend. Psychological distress tends to be somewhat less for survivors who are exposed to the disaster scene but not injured, persons who lose a more distant family member or friend, residents from the disaster zone whose homes were destroyed, rescue and recovery workers, and service providers working with bereaved survivors and their families. A proportion of mental health providers, clergy and chaplains, emergency health care professionals, government officials, and on-scene members of the media are also affected. More numerous, but less impacted, are groups that identify with the target-victim group, community businesses, and the community at large. These tiers of differential exposure to the traumatic effects of disaster are explored further in the following subsections to clarify how children feature prominently across this spectrum.

Direct Impact Survivors

For children, the severity of psychological distress and psychopathology, including posttraumatic stress symptoms, relates directly to their proximity to the zone of impact. The effects from being direct impact survivors have been documented in research spanning decades and including

TABLE 3–2.   **Factors that shape psychosocial responses to disasters**

Exposure factors	**Individual factors**
Intensity and duration of exposure	Age
	Gender
Direct involvement in the disaster	Level of cognitive and maturational development
Separation from loved ones and caretakers	History of separation or separation anxiety
Witnessing of event	Predisaster presence of psychopathology
Knowing someone who was injured or killed	History of exposure to traumatic events
Personal injury	
Exposure to brutal death and gruesome scenes	Subjective appraisal of the stressor
	Social support
Degree of life threat	Ability to elicit and use caretaker support
Child's subjective experience at the time of exposure	Predisaster and current adaptive and coping skills
Exposure through the media	
Family factors	**Community and societal factors**
Parental response	School community
Parent symptom choice	Social support networks
Family atmosphere	Community socioeconomic status
Communication patterns	Political structure and governance
Parental overprotectiveness	Culture/ethnicity
Separation from parents and siblings	
Prohibitive response to regression	
Reversal of the dependency role	

a remarkable diversity of incidents. As examples, the highest rates of posttraumatic stress symptoms were found for those children who were

- Inside a movie theater that was hit by a tornado (Bloch et al. 1956);
- Closest to a jungle gym on the playground where a child was killed during a school shooting (Pynoos et al. 1987);
- In the immediate path of raging Australian bush fires (McFarlane 1987);
- Closest to the eyewall of Hurricane Andrew, where the strongest winds were (Shaw et al. 1995, 1996);

- Trapped in attics and stranded in flood zones during Hurricane Katrina, including those children who believed they were going to die, who were physically injured, who lost their homes and were displaced, who lost a parent or family member to death from Katrina, and who were separated from parents and caregivers during and after the storm; and
- Exposed to missile attacks in southern Israel, compared with same-age counterparts in California (Wolmer et al. 2011).

Direct Witnesses

Direct witnesses are firsthand, frontline visual observers of harm who remarkably escape personal injury and do not sustain property loss or death of a family member or close friend. Adults and children who directly observed the collapse of the World Trade Center towers on September 11, 2001, and those who saw persons leaping from the upper floors of the towers were direct witnesses.

Indirectly Exposed Children

Children who were physically distant from the site of a disaster, but whose family members or friends were on the scene and were injured, killed, or traumatized, would be classified as indirectly exposed. These children are also at risk for psychological trauma based on this vicarious exposure.

Disaster Responders

The category of disaster responders includes first responders, rescue and recovery personnel, emergency health care service providers, government officials, members of the media, and mental health professionals. Although professional responders are adults, the relevance for children is evident: first responders are also parents, family members, or close friends of children. Moreover, children may bear witness, through media viewing, to the physical fatigue and psychological toll exacted from responders as they fulfill their duties. For children whose relatives are responding, these observations will be made directly, on the home front.

Disaster survivors and disaster responders alike are affected psychologically during extreme events. First responders are occupationally vulnerable to psychological impact. Responders at the disaster scene are met with a cacophonous, multisensory fusillade of images, sounds, smells, and sensations. They see the horrors of victims entrapped beyond the reach of rescue, and they attempt to accommodate the seemingly overwhelming waves of casualties in a catastrophic event.

Community at Large

Some disasters are focal in nature, whereas others have regional, national, or even international significance. For example, posttraumatic symptom expression was not restricted to those who were directly exposed to the 9/11 attack in lower Manhattan. Hundreds of thousands of residents of the New York City boroughs who were a safe distance from the scene were only indirectly exposed but were nevertheless psychologically affected (Galea and Resnick 2005). Moreover, the ripples of psychological effect were not confined to New York City; a nationwide survey of children ages 5–18 years, conducted 3–5 days after the 9/11 attack, found that 35% reported at least one symptom of posttraumatic stress, such as irritability, nightmares, avoiding hearing or talking about what happened, sleep problems, or trouble concentrating (Schuster et al. 2001). A survey of 8,266 children in grades 4–12, conducted by the New York City Department of Health and Mental Hygiene, indicated that following the attacks, rates of posttraumatic stress disorder (PTSD) increased fivefold from baseline, separation anxiety disorder doubled, and agoraphobia tripled (Fremont 2004).

Vicarious exposure to disasters via television and media coverage may also create psychological distress and impairment. Television viewing is a particularly powerful source of indirect exposure (Pfefferbaum et al. 2001; Schuster et al. 2001). Routine television viewing of traumatic situations can generate fear reactions and sleep disturbances among preschoolers and children of elementary school age. Emotional, behavioral, and stress-related symptoms have been repeatedly found in studies of children who were exposed to televised coverage of such traumatic events as the *Challenger* space shuttle explosion (Terr et al. 1999), the Oklahoma City bombing (Pfefferbaum et al. 2001), and the 9/11 terrorist attack on the World Trade Center.

Individual Factors

The effects of trauma on children and adolescents are mediated by a series of child-specific factors. As listed in Table 3–2, these factors include the child's age, gender, level of cognitive and maturational development, history of psychiatric disorders, prior exposure to traumatic events, primary coping styles, and ability to elicit and use caretaker support

(Pine and Cohen 2002). Additional factors that come into play when a disaster occurs include the child's subjective appraisal of the stressors associated with the event and the effectiveness of the child's capability to adapt and cope with the disaster and the associated hardships. Some of these factors are discussed in the following subsections.

Gender Differences

Boys are more likely than girls to be exposed to traumatic events. However, when exposed to trauma, girls are more likely to manifest anxiety and mood symptoms and to meet diagnostic criteria for PTSD (Green et al. 1991; Pine and Cohen 2002; Shaw et al. 1995, 1996). Shaw et al. (1996) found that after Hurricane Andrew, boys recovered more quickly from PTSD than did girls, but that boys manifested more disruptive behaviors.

Gender differences have also emerged in studies of children's responses to war-related trauma. For example, girls exposed to armed conflict in Croatia displayed more symptoms of anxiety and depression than did boys similarly exposed, whereas boys manifested a lower level of psychosocial adaptation (Vizek-Vidovic et al. 2000).

Preexisting Psychopathology

Children with a history of emotional and behavioral problems (particularly anxiety disorders), cognitive impairment, learning disorders, separation anxiety, or depression are at higher risk for psychological consequences following disasters.

Prior Trauma Exposure

In contrast to the philosopher Friedrich Nietzsche's aphorism, "That which does not kill us makes us stronger," the reality is that trauma exposure usually does not have a protective inoculation effect. To the contrary, repeated trauma exposure tends to produce a cumulative detrimental effect, with loss of resilience and increased vulnerability to future trauma exposure. The prior exposure of children to trauma is associated with higher risks for psychopathology when they experience later traumatic events.

Subjective Appraisal

A survivor's subjective appraisal of a disaster or traumatic experience also relates to the occurrence of adverse psychological effects. How the individual defines the traumatic situation and what meaning he or she imposes on the event are strong predictors of outcome. A person's perception of a traumatic situation at the time of exposure is a mediator of psychological response. For adolescents on the sinking cruise ship *Jupiter*, predictors of posttraumatic symptomatology were thinking that they would not escape, panic feelings, and fear of imminent death (Udwin et al. 2000). The most prevalent and distressing subjective appraisals reported by middle school children following the Oklahoma City bombing were fears that a family member or friend would be hurt, and feeling nervous and afraid (Pfefferbaum et al. 2002). In the latter study, these peritraumatic responses were even more strongly associated with psychopathological outcomes than were immediate physical exposure, relatedness to a victim of the bombing, or repetitive television viewing of the incident.

Family Factors

The reactions that a disaster evokes from the family caregivers will be telegraphed to the children (Green et al. 1991; McFarlane 1987; Shaw 2000, 2003). The family's critical role as caretaker for children will be detrimentally affected when parents are emotionally distressed and will be frankly compromised in situations of disaster-related parental death, injury, illness, or separation from the children.

Children frequently mirror the fears, anxieties, and symptom choices exhibited by their parents as a disaster or other traumatic event is unfolding. Levels of psychological distress in children can be predicted based on their observations of their parents' reactions and coping strategies while a disaster is striking. Elevated risks for children are associated with disaster-related parental psychopathology, negative family emotional tone, distressed family environment, parental overprotectiveness, reversal of the dependency role, and excessive prohibition of regressive behaviors (Shaw 2000). McFarlane (1987), for example, found that the mother's psychological response to an Australian bushfire disaster was a better predictor of the child's psychological well-being than was the child's direct exposure.

On the basis of these findings, mental health professionals generally accept that the presence of parental psychopathology and family dysfunction in response to traumatic events predicts higher levels of psychological morbidity in children. The research literature on war and armed conflict provides further support for this contention. For example, the psychological response of Lebanese children, ages 5–7 years, who were exposed to war-related trauma was best predicted by the level of depres-

TABLE 3–3. Family stressors

Predisaster	Postdisaster
Family atmosphere	Parent symptom choice
Parental psychopathology	Separation from parents, caretakers, or siblings
Overprotectiveness	
Dysfunctional parents	Prohibitive response to regression
Marital instability	Reversal of the dependency role
Single-parent household	Multiple stressors (loss of home; property and financial loss)
Low socioeconomic status	
Family history of neuroticism (proneness to experience irritability, depression, and anxiety)	Prolonged displacement
	Continued separation and estrangement from family and friends
	Resource deterioration
	Marital distress
	Decline in perceived social support
	Financial distress (unemployment)

sive symptoms in their mothers (Bryce et al. 1989). The findings from research conducted on the reactions of children exposed to war-related trauma provide insights into children's reactions to disaster. War, which undermines a child's sense of security, has a devastating and enduring effect on the family and the social fabric of a community. Family factors, mediated by social contexts such as displacement, play a crucial role in shaping the child's psychological response to war-related situations. Indeed, contextual factors interact with war-related traumas as a mediator of children's psychological response. Almqvist and Broberg (1999) found that the degree of family support predicts children's long-term emotional response to being a refugee. Higher rates of psychological morbidity were found among displaced Israeli families than among nondisplaced families with comparable levels of exposure to the Scud missile attacks during the 1991 Gulf War (Laor et al. 2001).

Other family features that negatively influence psychological outcomes for children are marital conflict and instability, low socioeconomic status, family history of neuroticism, and single-parent households. Conversely, the existence of parental and family support mitigates the risk for posttraumatic stress symptoms. Family stressors before and after disaster are summarized in Table 3–3.

TABLE 3–4.   **Community and societal stressors**

Predisaster	Postdisaster
Family atmosphere	Loss of community infrastructure
Level of preparedness	Resource deterioration
Lack of emergency management system resources	Loss of health care services
	Social support deterioration
Poverty	Media attention
Lack of civil government leadership	Closure of schools
	Perceived or actual failure of
Ethnic and racial disparities	government response

Community and Societal Factors

Community refers to a social context with its network of relationships, but more importantly, it refers to shared values, understandings, and a common outlook regarding what is important in life. A number of authors have observed the devastating psychological effects of disaster on a community and the ever-widening circles of involvement, beginning with directly exposed individuals and moving outward to family members, friends, neighbors, first responders, and the surrounding community of individuals who are distressed and suffer vicariously (Erikson 1976; Taylor and Fraser 1981; Wright et al. 1990). The child's psychological vulnerability mimics that of the community at large. Community disruption generates a broad composite of secondary stressors that may affect a child (Table 3–4). One important disaster-related community disruption that represents a significant adversity for children is the impact on the school community, marked by school closures, interrupted or canceled youth activities, and emotionally distressed teachers and staff (many of whom are also survivors) (Pynoos et al. 1998). Community and societal stressors before and after the disaster are noted in Table 3–4.

In a disaster, the *impact ratio,* calculated as the proportion of disaster victims to total citizens in a disaster-affected community, is a useful metric to consider as a community-level indicator of psychosocial outcomes following a disaster. In a study of 10 eastern Kentucky counties affected by widespread flooding, the impact ratio consistently predicted rates of depression, anxiety, and somatic symptoms after controlling for the effects of personal loss. Counties that fared most poorly were those with high levels of personal loss for many citizens in combination with extensive neighborhood destruction. The capacity of a community of disaster survivors to cope and recover pivots on a cluster of synergistic factors that collectively define the community's "social surround," including social support, socioeconomic status, political structure, governance, and culture/ethnicity (Somasundaram et al. 2003).

A high proportion of individuals (estimates range from 25% to 75%) in the disaster impact zone will experience a significant stress response that will temporarily compromise functioning during the impact and rescue phases. A substantial minority will progress from initial distress to significant psychological morbidity in the year following disaster (World Health Organization 1992). Alexander et al. (2004) suggested that in some instances, the effects of the disaster are so far-reaching that the catastrophic impact will fundamentally transform the community at large. Archetypal examples of humanitarian catastrophes include Hiroshima, the Holocaust, the 9/11 attacks, the 2004 Southeast Asia tsunami, and the 2010 Haiti earthquake. Alexander et al. (2004) further suggested that a cultural trauma has occurred when members of a community have been so affected that future group identity is impacted in a "fundamental and irrevocable" manner. The effects will be multigenerational, and trauma will be transmitted intergenerationally.

Social and Community Support

Each child and family unit as a whole is affected by the quality of social supports and social infrastructure. Disasters may produce devastating effects on available social supports through breakdown of communication channels, displacement of populations, separation of loved ones, large-scale mortality, and debilitating injury. Closure of schools and community programs where children congregate will decrease access to usual sources of socialization and peer support. Somasundaram et al. (2003) observed that following a disaster, victims may have difficulty maintaining supportive relationships just when most needed. Exacerbating this situation, increased rates of divorce and family violence have been reported after some disasters. Disaster recovery, a challenging period for all families, is even more difficult for families of minority status, single-parent families, families supporting persons with special needs, and displaced or refugee families (Shaw et al. 2007).

Socioeconomic Status and Poverty

The unfavorable association between poverty and mental health has been described worldwide throughout history (Costello et al. 2003). Socioeconomic disadvantage negatively affects children's mental health and is related to decreased intelligence, academic achievement, and social and emotional functioning (Gilliam et al. 2007). Family and neighborhood poverty is associated with an impoverished home environment and less parental warmth. Behavior problems such as disobedience, interpersonal conflict, and rule violations are more prevalent for children in households with low socioeconomic status (Achenbach et al. 1987). These negative influences of socioeconomic disadvantage on child behavior are mediated by chronic exposure to stress and uncertainty and by dysfunctional parenting practices that are harsh, punitive, inconsistent, and unsupportive (Boyle and Lipman 2002).

In addition, empirical data suggest that children from low-income families are more likely to have chronic illnesses, mental health problems, and disabilities than are their more affluent counterparts (Brooks-Gunn and Duncan 1997), yet are less likely to have a regular source of medical care and preventive health care services (Oberg et al. 1995). An inverse relationship exists between household income and emotional and behavioral problems in childhood (Gilliam et al. 2007). In general, poor children are more likely to exhibit anxiety, social withdrawal, depression, and disruptive behaviors than are children from economically stable families (Duncan et al. 1994). Persistent poverty is more harmful to children's mental health than is transient poverty because of greater economic deprivation (Brooks-Gunn and Duncan 1997; Mcleod and Shanahan 1996). This complex substrate of vulnerability factors is already operating when disaster strikes children in poverty.

Disasters invariably diminish the economic stability and viability of a community. Workplaces are destroyed, transportation and communication systems are damaged, unemployment increases, and financial resources must be redirected to fund response and recovery. Low-income households as well as entire low-income communities tend to populate hazardous locales that offer minimal citizen protection and disaster mitigation resources. When a disaster occurs, these families are more vulnerable to its consequences than are families with greater means.

In a review of studies on the relationship between poverty and disasters in the United States, Fothergill and Peek (2004) reported that socioeconomic status is a significant determinant of the severity of both physical and psychological disaster consequences. Before a disaster, poor families were more likely to display higher rates of mental illness and mental health risk factors. During disaster, they were more likely to experience psychiatric and psychological symptoms, physical injury, death, and extensive damage to dwellings. These hardships were exacerbated in the aftermath because these families were likely to encounter more obstacles during disaster response, recovery, and reconstruction.

When Hurricane Katrina struck New Orleans, 38% of children under age 18 years were below the poverty level, including 17,000 children below age 6 (Golden 2006). Many children (40%) were separated from family members during the disaster but knew where they were; 13% were separated and did not know where their families were located. Among children separated from family members, those living in poverty were disproportionately represented.

Geography

Patterns of human settlement and quality of housing construction both play a role in determining vulnerability to disasters. Prior to Hurricane Katrina's impact, certain areas within New Orleans could be identified geographically as high-stress environments for families and youth based on limited employment opportunities, low educational attainment, high crime rates, and poor health indicators (Curtis et al. 2007). These areas indeed had the most vulnerable housing and sustained the greatest disaster-related physical destruction, loss of life, injury, population displacement, interpersonal violence, and looting. Because of their ongoing high-hazard, high-vulnerability potential, some of the hardest-hit areas have not been repopulated. Many former residents have been broadly dispersed, and some of these communities have ceased to exist. In summary, the convergence of multiple ecological, social, political, and economic risk factors, all overlapping within a definable geographic area, led to high rates of mortality, injury, physical illness, and psychological impairment for these residents (Walker and Warren 2007).

Political Structure and Governance

Response and intervention following disaster exposure are influenced by political structure and governance. Disaster-affected local municipalities may want to tap the available national or state resources and expertise while simultaneously resenting and resisting what they perceive to be intrusion into their jurisdiction.

Much of the impact of Hurricane Katrina on children reflected shortcomings in the planning and governance process (Dolan and Krug 2006). Absence of viable evacuation strategies left many children unnecessarily in harm's way during the storm. The evacuation process that was improvised in the aftermath frequently separated children from parents and caregivers, yet no effective mechanisms were in place for reuniting children with their parents. The situation was most egregious for separated infants and preverbal toddlers whose identities could not be readily confirmed to assure proper placement. The government was unable to support children's health care services. The complete lack of mental health interventions for children affected by the hurricane, resources for non-English-speaking children, and customized care for children with special medical needs contributed to increased rates of death, injury, and psychiatric morbidity (Dolan and Krug 2006).

Culture/Ethnicity

As defined by Wseng (2003), *culture* is "the unique behavior patterns and lifestyle shared by a group of people, which distinguish it from others" (p. 5), whereas *ethnicity* refers to "social groups that distinguish themselves from other groups by a common historical path, behavior norms, and their own group identities" (p. 7). To achieve further clarification, Wseng asserts that "culture refers to manifest characteristic behavior patterns and value systems, whereas ethnicity refers to a group of people that share a common feature or root culture" (p. 8).

Disaster is a social experience. Cultural groups, particularly those representing minorities or recent immigrants, experience the full range of disaster stressors, compounded by these additional stressors: language difficulties, lack of insurance, limited financial resources, discrimination from members of other cultural groups, unfamiliarity with community support systems, difficulty accessing disaster services, and immigration status issues. Recent immigrants may lack understanding of the systems of help that are available in their adopted culture. Members of some cultural groups are both marginalized and impoverished—a synergistic combination that amplifies their vulnerability to the destructive forces of disaster. In disasters, ethnic minorities experience more adverse psychological consequences than do members of the majority culture (Norris and Alegria 2005). Disadvantaged and minority populations have a higher rate and greater intensity of exposure to predisaster trauma and are more vulnerable to subsequent trauma when disaster strikes (Breslau et al. 1998). In fact, ethnic communities face increased vulnerability to disaster hazards across all disaster phases: risk perception, preparedness, warning, physical impact, psychological impact, rescue, recovery, and reconstruction (Fothergill et al. 1999). These findings prompted Cutter (2006) to assert, "Disasters are income neutral and color-blind. Their impacts, however, are not." Risk disparities for ethnic minorities by disaster phases are listed in Table 3–5.

TABLE 3–5.   **Risk disparities for ethnic minorities, by disaster stage**

Disaster stage	Impact on ethnic minorities
Preparedness behavior	Preparedness behavior stage of the disaster life cycle encompasses all preparation activities and mitigation efforts in advance of a specific warning. Potential preparedness risks for ethnic minorities: Lack of information in native language Lack of financial resources to obtain preparedness materials Living in areas more vulnerable to damage from disaster hazards
Warning communication and response	Warning communication and response stage entails receiving warnings or other risk communications regarding an immediate danger and taking some type of action, such as evacuation, in response to this warning. Potential warning communication and response risks for ethnic minorities: Lack of information in native language Lack of transportation Evacuation difficulties
Physical impact	Physical impact stage is concerned with the actual and immediate effects of the disaster striking a community. Physical impacts include mortality, morbidity and injury rates, as well as economic losses. Often, these rates are directly related to safe housing. Potential physical impact risks for ethnic minorities: Housing that is structurally unsafe
Emergency response	Emergency response stage occurs in the immediate aftermath of the disaster. Emergency response risks for ethnic minorities: Cultural insensitivity of emergency personnel Limited access of responders to victims Lack of information Immigration status as a barrier to seeking and receiving benefits Language difficulties

TABLE 3–5.	Risk disparities for ethnic minorities, by disaster stage *(continued)*
Disaster stage	Impact on ethnic minorities
Recovery	Recovery stage refers to the first full year following a disaster.
	Potential recovery risks for ethnic minorities: Lower incomes, lower savings account balances, greater unemployment, less property insurance, and less access to communication channels and information Lack of health insurance Difficulty accessing disaster services and navigating bureaucracies
Reconstruction	Reconstruction stage follows recovery, extending several years beyond the disaster. Reconstruction surrounds a community's long-term restoration, including rebuilding, replacing infrastructure, obtaining loans, receiving assistance, and locating permanent housing.
	Potential reconstruction risks for ethnic minorities: Physical displacement Stigmatization of the affected area Decline in standards of living Loss of community and jobs Economic decline

Among children, ethnicity has been found to shape psychological outcomes following disasters. In an exhaustive review of the disaster literature, Norris et al. (2002) found four studies in which minority youth fared worse than majority youth (Garrison et al. 1993; La Greca et al. 1998; March et al. 1997; Shannon et al. 1994) and two studies in which the minority youth fared better (Garrison et al. 1993; Jones et al. 2001). Lengua et al. (2005) studied the psychological response of children following the 9/11 attacks, and noted that African American children reported more avoidant posttraumatic stress symptoms and feelings of upset than did Caucasian children.

■ Key Clinical Points

- ■ Disaster results in both psychosocial and ecological disruption of the community.

- ■ The disaster ecology model portrays disaster as the encounter between forces of harm and the human population.

- ■ The disaster ecology model assumes that there are gradations of human exposure to the traumatizing effects of disaster.

- ■ The child's psychological response to disaster is influenced by contextual factors within the child's environment.

- ■ Psychological morbidity is affected by the intensity of disaster exposure and social connectedness to directly impacted victims.

- ■ Community and societal factors, such as culture/ethnicity, poverty, minority status, geography, and governance, influence the survivors' psychological responses to disaster.

References

Achenbach TM, Verhulst FC, Edelbrock C, et al: Epidemiological comparisons of American and Dutch children, II: behavioral/emotional problems reported by teachers for ages 6 to 11. J Am Acad Child Adolesc Psychiatry 26:326–332, 1987

Alexander JC, Eyerman R, Giesen B, et al: Cultural Trauma and Collective Identity. Berkeley, University of California Press, 2004

Almqvist K, Broberg AG: Mental health and social adjustment in young refugee children 3 1/2 years after their arrival in Sweden. J Am Acad Child Adolesc Psychiatry 38:723–730, 1999

Bloch D, Silber E, Perry S: Some factors in the emotional reactions of children to disaster. Am J Psychiatry 113:416–422, 1956

Boyle MH, Lipman EL: Do places matter? Socioeconomic disadvantage and behavioral problems of children in Canada. J Consult Clin Psychology 70:378–389, 2002

Breslau N, Kessler RC, Chilcoat HD, et al: Trauma and posttraumatic stress disorder in the community: the 1996 Detroit Area Survey of Trauma. Arch Gen Psychiatry 55:626–632, 1998

Brooks-Gunn J, Duncan GJ: The effects of poverty on children. Future Child 7:55–71, 1997

Bryce JW, Walker N, Ghorayeb F, et al: Life experiences, response styles and mental health among mothers and children in Beirut, Lebanon. Soc Sci Med 28:685–695, 1989

Costello EJ, Compton SN, Keeler G, et al: Relationships between poverty and psychopathology: a natural experiment. JAMA 290:2023–2029, 2003

Curtis A, Mills JW, Leitner M: Katrina and vulnerability: the geography of stress. J Health Care Poor Underserved 18:315–330, 2007

Cuttler S: The Geography of Social Vulnerability: Race, Class, and Catastrophe. June 11, 2006. Available at: http://understandingkatrina.ssrc.org/Cutter. Accessed August 22, 2011.

Dolan MA, Krug SE: Pediatric disaster preparedness in the wake of Katrina: lessons to be learned. Clin Pediatr Emerg Med 7:59–66, 2006

Duncan GJ, Brook-Gunn J, Klebanov PK: Economic deprivation and early child development. Child Dev 65 (2, spec no):296–318, 1994

Erikson K: Disaster at Buffalo Creek: loss of communality at Buffalo Creek. Am J Psychiatry 133:302–305, 1976

Fothergill A, Peek L: Poverty and disasters in the United States: a review of recent sociological findings. Natural Hazards 32:89–110, 2004

Fothergill A, Maestas EG, Darlington JD: Race, ethnicity and disasters in the United Status: a review of the literature. Disasters 23:156–173, 1999

Fremont W: Childhood reactions to terrorism-induced trauma: a review of the past 10 years. J Am Acad Child Adolesc Psychiatry 43:381–392, 2004

Galea S, Resnick H: Posttraumatic stress disorder in the general population after mass terrorist incidents: considerations about the nature of exposure. CNS Spectr 10:107–115, 2005

Garrison CZ, Weinrich MW, Hardin SB, et al: Post-traumatic stress disorder in adolescents after a hurricane. Am J Epidemiol 138:522–530, 1993

Gilliam WS, Zigler EF, Finn-Stevenson M: Child and family policy: a role for child psychiatry and allied disciplines, in Lewis's Child and Adolescent Psychiatry. Edited by Martin A, Volkmar FR. Philadelphia, PA, Wolters Kluwer, 2007, pp 33–56

Golden O: Young children after Katrina: a proposal to heal the damage and create opportunity in New Orleans, in After Katrina: Rebuilding Opportunity and Equity Into the *New* New Orleans. Washington, DC, The Urban Institute. February 2006. Available at: http://www.urban.org/publications/900920.html. Accessed August 22, 2011.

Green BL, Korol M, Grace MC, et al: Children and disaster: age, gender and parental effects on PTSD symptoms. J Am Acad Child Adolesc Psychiatry 30:945–951, 1991

Jones RT, Frary R, Cunningham P, et al: The psychological effects of Hurricane Andrew on ethnic minority and Caucasian children and adolescents: a case study. Cultur Divers Ethnic Minor Psychol 7:103–108, 2001

La Greca AM, Silverman WK, Wasserstein SB: Children's pre-disaster functioning as a predictor of posttraumatic stress following Hurricane Andrew. J Consult Clin Psychol 66:883–892, 1998

Laor N, Wolmer L, Cohen DJ: Mothers' functioning and children's symptoms 5 years after a SCUD missile attack. Am J Psychiatry 158:1020–1026, 2001

Lengua LJ, Long AC, Smith KL, et al: Pre-attack symptomatology and temperament as predictors of children's responses to the September 11 terrorist attacks. J Child Psychol Psychiatry 46:631–645, 2005

March JS, Amaya-Jackson L, Terry R, et al: Posttraumatic symptomatology in children and adolescents after an industrial fire. J Am Acad Child Adolesc Psychiatry 36:1080–1088, 1997

McFarlane AC: Posttraumatic phenomena in a longitudinal study of children following a natural disaster. J Am Acad Child Adolesc Psychiatry 26:764–769, 1987

Mcleod JD, Shanahan MJ: Trajectories of poverty and children's mental health. J Health Soc Behav 37:207–220, 1996

Norris FH, Alegria M: Mental health care for ethnic minority individuals and communities in the aftermath of disasters and mass violence. CNS Spectr 10:132–140, 2005

Norris FH, Friedman MJ, Watson PJ: 60,000 disaster victims speak, part 1: an empirical review of the empirical literature. Psychiatry 65:207–239, 2002

Oberg CN, Bryant NA, Bach ML: A portrait of America's children: the impact of poverty and a call to action. Journal of Social Distress and the Homeless 4:43–56, 1995

Pfefferbaum B, Nixon SJ, Tivis RD, et al: Television exposure in children after a terrorist incident. Psychiatry 64:202–211, 2001

Pfefferbaum B, Doughty DE, Reddy C, et al: Exposure and peritraumatic response as predictors of posttraumatic stress in children following the 1995 Oklahoma City bombing. J Urban Health 79:354–363, 2002

Pine OS, Cohen JA: Trauma in children and adolescents: risk and treatment of psychiatric sequelae. Biol Psychiatry 51:519–531, 2002

Pynoos RS, Frederick C, Nader K, et al: Life threat and posttraumatic stress in school-age children. Arch Gen Psychiatry 44:1057–1063, 1987

Pynoos RS, Goenjian AK, Steinberg AM: A public mental health approach to the postdisaster treatment of children and adolescents. Child Adolesc Psychiatr Clin N Am 7:195–210, 1998

Schuster MA, Stein BD, Jaycox L, et al: A national survey of stress reactions after the September 11, 2001, terrorist attacks. New Engl J Med 345:1507–1512, 2001

Shannon MP, Lonigan CJ, Finch AJ, et al: Children exposed to disaster, epidemiology of post-traumatic symptoms and symptom profile. J Am Acad Child Adolesc Psychiatry 33:80–93, 1994

Shaw JA: Children, adolescents and trauma. Psychiatr Q 71:227–234, 2000

Shaw JA: Children exposed to war/terrorism. Clin Child Fam Psychol Rev 6:237–246, 2003

Shaw JA, Applegate B, Tanner S, et al: Psychological effects of Hurricane Andrew on an elementary school population. J Am Acad Child Adolesc Psychiatry 34:1185–1192, 1995

Shaw JA, Applegate B, Schorr C: Twenty-one-month follow-up study of school-age children exposed to Hurricane Andrew. J Am Acad Child Adolesc Psychiatry 35:359–364, 1996

Shaw JA, Espinel Z, Shultz JM: Children: Stress, Trauma and Disasters. Tampa, FL, Disaster Life Support Publishing, 2007

Shultz JM, Espinel Z, Flynn BW, et al: All-Hazards Disaster Behavioral Health Training. Tampa, FL, Disaster Life Support Publishing, 2007

Somasundaram D, Norris FH, Asukai N, et al: Natural and technological disasters, in Trauma Interventions in War and Peace: Prevention, Practice and Policy. Edited by Green BL, Friedman MJ, de Jong JT, et al. New York, Kluwer Academic/Plenum, 2003, pp 291–318

Taylor AJW, Fraser AG: Psychological Sequelae of Operation Overdue Following the DC-10 Aircrash in Antarctica (Victoria University of Wellington Publications in Psychology No 27). Wellington, New Zealand, Victoria University, 1981

Terr LC, Bloch DA, Michel BA, et al: Children's symptoms in the wake of Challenger: a field study of distant-traumatic effects and an outline of related conditions. Am J Psychiatry 156:1536–1544, 1999

Udwin O, Boyle S, Yule W, et al: Risk factors for long-term psychological effects of a disaster experienced in adolescence: predictors of post traumatic stress disorder. J Child Psychol Psychiatry 41:969–979, 2000

Vizek-Vidovic V, Kuterovac-Jagodic G, Arambasic L: Posttraumatic symptomatology in children exposed to war. Scand J Psychol 41:297–306, 2000

Walker B, Warren RC: Katrina perspectives. J Health Care Poor Underserved 18:233–240, 2007

Wolmer L, Hamiel D, Loar N: Preventing children's posttraumatic stress after disaster with teacher-based intervention: a controlled study. J Am Acad Child Adolesc Psychiatry 50:340–348, 2011

World Health Organization, Division of Mental Health: Psychosocial Consequences of Disaster: Prevention and Management. Geneva, World Health Organization, 1992

Wright KM, Ursano RJ, Bartone PT, et al: The shared experience of catastrophe: an expanded classificatiion of the disaster community. Am J Orthopsychiatry 60:35–42, 1990

Wseng WS: Clinician's Guide to Cultural Psychiatry. San Diego, CA, Academic Press, 2003

4

Children's Psychological Responses to Disasters

Introduction

Children are particularly vulnerable to the effects of traumatic events because they lack the experience, skills, and individual resources to independently meet their mental and behavioral health needs (National Commission on Children and Disasters 2010). The National Commission on Children and Disasters (2010) has noted the unique needs of children exposed to disasters and the importance of viewing children as more than just small adults (Table 4–1).

TABLE 4–1.   Children's unique needs in disasters

Children may experience long-lasting effects such as academic failure, posttraumatic stress disorder, depression, anxiety, bereavement, and other behavioral problems such as delinquency and substance abuse.

Children are more susceptible to chemical, biological, radiological, and nuclear threats and require different medications, dosages, and delivery systems than adults.

During disasters, young children may not be able escape danger, identify themselves, and make critical decisions.

Children are dependent on adults for care, shelter, transportation, and protection from predators.

Children are often away from parents, in the care of schools, child care providers, Head Start, or other child congregate care environments, which must be prepared to ensure children's safety.

Children must be expeditiously reunified with their legal guardians if separated from them during a disaster.

Children in disaster shelters require age-appropriate supplies such as diapers, cribs, baby formula, and food.

Source.   Reprinted from National Commission on Children and Disasters: *2010 Report to the President and Congress* (AHRQ Publ. No. 10-M037). Rockville, MD, Agency for Healthcare Research and Quality, October 2010. Available at: http://www. acf.hhs.gov/ohsepr/nccdreport. Accessed August 25, 2011.

A child's psychological response to trauma is fundamentally affected by his or her level of cognitive and emotional development and the family context. The child typically lives within a family system that is integrated into a community within a larger cultural and ethnic group. The child's responses to disaster are influenced by the family ambience; the psychological responses of parents, family members, and other members of the community; and the family's response to the perceived increased dependency needs of their children impacted by disaster (Hoven et al. 2009).

Independent of the specific type of trauma, psychological responses tend to follow several common pathways (Figure 4–1). Life threat and the threat of physical injury may result in psychological distress manifested by posttraumatic stress symptoms; grief and depression may occur secondary to losses; anxiety symptoms may result from worrying about self and others; and ongoing stressors may cause behavioral problems to develop (Pynoos and Nader 1988). Children with preexisting emotional and behavioral problems may experience exacerbation of symptoms

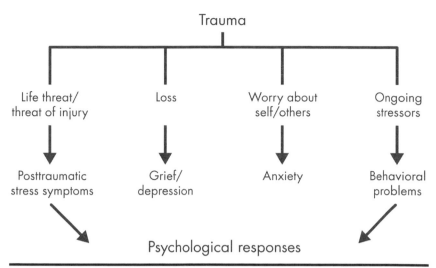

FIGURE 4–1.   Spectrum of psychological responses to trauma.

Source.   Adapted from Pynoos and Nader 1988.

following disaster, particularly when critical medications are in short supply and when social supports diminish and routines are disrupted. Children with physical illness may find that the postdisaster demands overwhelm their precarious coping capacities. Following the disaster-related death of a parent or a family member, children may experience traumatic bereavement.

Developmental Effects

A child's psychological response is determined and shaped not only by the nature of the disaster but also by the child's level of cognitive development, egocentric theories of causality, personality characteristics, and biological resilience; reactions of family members; and the effectiveness of the child's adaptive and coping mechanisms for regulating mood and emotions.

Preschool Children

Preschool children are less likely to experience posttraumatic symptoms than are older children (Bloch et al. 1956; Green et al. 1991). Younger children rely on parental and family figures to determine their perceived degree of risk or safety. Children often mirror parents' emotional states,

---

TABLE 4–2.   Psychological responses of preschool children to disasters

---

Sleep and appetite disturbances

Clinging and dependent behavior

Separation anxiety

Fear of the dark

Nightmares

Disorganized and regressive behaviors

Hypervigilance

Behavioral reenactments

---

attitudes, and behaviors. As long as parents respond with some sense of equanimity, children often feel protected and secure. Younger children have less specific cognitive awareness regarding the nature and meaning of a traumatic experience. Reactions of preschool children tend to be disorganized and agitated, manifested by generalized fears, separation anxiety, aggressive and disruptive behaviors, physical complaints, or loss of previously mastered bowel and bladder control.

A child's level of cognitive development has a profound effect on the child's interpretation of and psychological response to a traumatic situation. Piaget (1967) observed that children do not recognize the existence of chance happenings and believe that everything that happens is related to something they did or did not do. A child may interpret a trauma as a punishment for a self-perceived transgression. One child who was evacuated to a shelter because of extensive flooding in his hometown believed the floods were a direct consequence of his repeatedly flushing the toilet at home, a behavior for which he had been reprimanded. A young girl believed that the Chowchilla, California, bus kidnapping had occurred because she had called her mother "the meanest mother in the world" as she left for school that morning (Terr 1981b). A child in Miami thought that Hurricane Andrew had occurred because he hit his brother.

Younger children often have a skewed sense of time and have difficulty placing events in chronological order. Children may be prone to illusory experiences and cognitive distortions as they recount their traumatic experiences. They may embellish or fabricate missing explanatory pieces from their own fears and wishes. Terr (1988) noted that preschool children under age 3 years have little capacity to verbally recall their traumatic experiences, although girls are generally more suc-

TABLE 4–3.	Psychological responses of school-age children to disasters

Reexperiencing of symptoms

Disorganized or confused behaviors

Somatic complaints

Arousal symptoms

Disruptive behaviors

Anxiety symptoms

Decreased academic performance

cessful than boys. Younger children are more likely to reenact the trauma experience in their play activities and insert aspects of the disaster event into drawings or storytelling (Terr 1981a, 1991). Table 4–2 lists the psychological responses of preschool children.

School-Age Children

The school-age child has a more mature cognitive understanding of the nature of a disaster event or traumatic situation, including potential threats of bodily injury and death. Symptoms following disaster exposure may include disturbance of regular sleep patterns, appetite change, behavioral problems in school, decline in academic performance, disruptive behaviors, depression, anxiety disorders, somatic concerns, and symptoms of posttraumatic stress disorder (PTSD). School-age children may experience secondary psychological symptoms as a consequence of their hyperarousal, agitation, anxiety, or somatic symptoms. Table 4–3 lists the psychological responses in school-age children.

Adolescents

The Institute of Medicine (IOM) and National Research Council (NRC) (2011) define *adolescence* as that period of time that occurs between 10 and 19 years of age, and reported that adolescents constitute 14% of the population. The momentous changes that occur during puberty, the pruning of synaptic connections, and the postulated attenuation of mesolimbic dopamine activity contribute to a reward deficiency syndrome during adolescence that may lead to risk-taking or sensation-seeking behaviors and the abuse of alcohol or other substances (Spear 2007). Youth preoccupied with intrusive images, overwhelmed with traumatic reminders, or concerned with a foreshortened life have little energy to meet age-appropriate developmental tasks (National Child Traumatic Stress Network 2008).

As children emerge into adolescence, posttraumatic stress symptoms become more like the adult pattern, with a similar range of symptoms and clinical presentations. However, the psychological response is often colored by the adolescent's awareness of a life unlived. Exposure to a perceived threat to life and safety may precipitate fear of a foreshortened future, accentuating the sense of biological fragility and increasing awareness of life's transience (Shaw 2000). Subsequent to disaster, adolescents may avoid previously enjoyed activities or, alternatively, take flight into pleasure-seeking pursuits based on the sudden realization of life's potential brevity. Table 4–4 summarizes the psychological responses of adolescents.

Stress Reactions to Disasters

Acute Stress Responses

The majority of persons exposed to a life-threatening experience will manifest acute stress symptoms. During the disaster impact phase, children are often at risk for physical harm and even death. They can be expected to experience psychological distress from exposure to horrific happenings and witnessing harm to others. Most children and their families experience a normal stress response characterized by anxiety, fear, and feelings of helplessness; grief and mourning in response to losses; mood and anxiety symptoms associated with separation from friends and loved ones; behavioral problems; and somatic illnesses. In most instances, the stress symptoms dissipate as normal functioning is restored to the resilient child. In some instances, children may manifest an increasing incapacity to adapt to changing circumstances and may go on to meet criteria for a diagnosable mental disorder. This range of psychological responses to disaster is depicted in Figure 4–2.

Children and adolescents exposed to disasters exhibit acute stress responses in several domains of human functioning, including changes in physiology, behavior, mood, thinking, and interpersonal relationships. Table 4–5 itemizes common acute stress reactions in children and adolescents.

Following the destructive impact of a tornado striking Vicksburg, Mississippi, one-third of the children exhibited psychological reactions

TABLE 4–4.   **Psychological responses of adolescents to disasters**

Anxiety

Depression

Guilt, anger, fear, disillusionment

Fears of a foreshortened future

Changes in social behaviors

Flight into pleasurable pursuits

Substance abuse

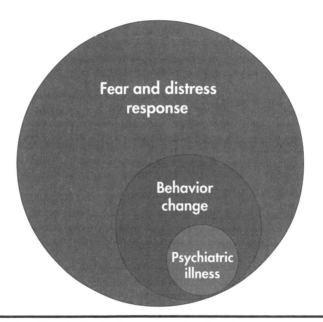

FIGURE 4–2.   **Psychological response to disaster.**
Source.   Institute of Medicine 2003.

that included anxiety, clinging and dependent behaviors, sleep disturbances, night terrors, and regressive behaviors (Bloch et al. 1956). Terr
(1981b) described the psychological effects of human-generated violence on children. During the 1976 Chowchilla bus kidnapping, 23 children, ages 5–14 years, were held captive on a school bus for 26 hours.
Following the episode, many of these children experienced traumatic
nightmares (50%), fears of recurrence (85%), posttraumatic play involving themes of kidnapping (55%), and cognitive disturbances.

TABLE 4–5.   Acute stress reactions in children and adolescents

Changes in bodily function	Somatic complaints: headaches, stomachaches
	Sleep and appetite disturbances
Changes in behavior	Disruptive behaviors
	Hyperactivity
	Clinging and dependent behaviors
	Avoidant and phobic symptoms
	Regressive behaviors
	Feelings of a foreshortened future
	Flight into pleasure-seeking activities
	Substance abuse
Changes in mood	Specific fears that the disaster will recur
	Feelings of insecurity, anxiety, fear, anger, sadness
	Irritability
	Feelings of unfairness
	Increased concerns regarding the safety of loved ones
Changes in thinking	Child's distorted belief that he or she has caused the disaster
	Loss of trust in the safety and security of the world
	Loss of trust in adults' ability to protect children
	Decreased concentration
Changes in interpersonal and social relationships	Social withdrawal
	Increased immersion into peer-related activities

Shaw et al. (1995) found that 87% of school-age children in the direct path of Hurricane Andrew had moderate to severe posttraumatic stress symptoms, and 57% had severe to very severe posttraumatic stress symptoms. The most common stress symptoms were sleep disturbances, nightmares, fears of recurrence, anxiety, and fears when thinking about the hurricane. Following the 2004 Indian Ocean tsunami, 14%–38% of children ages 8–14 years experienced posttraumatic stress symptoms

(Neuner et al. 2006). The prevalence and severity of symptoms were directly related to the intensity of the traumatic exposure. Following the September 11, 2001, attacks on America, a national survey found that 35% of children had one or more symptoms of stress and that 47% were concerned about their own safety (Schuster et al. 2001). Twenty-two percent of children in Manhattan were referred for counseling following the September 11 attack (Stuber et al. 2002).

Chronic Stress Responses

In the aftermath of disaster, a cascade of hardships and adversities (secondary stressors) continues to have an impact on the child and family. Following disaster, exposure to chronic stressors may progressively erode the child's resilience and increase the risk for psychological disorders and medical illnesses. Cumulative stress increases the risk for central nervous system changes, anxiety, depression, dissociative reactions, suicidal thoughts, personality changes, substance abuse, loss and grief reactions, decreased social function, and aggressive and delinquent behaviors.

In a study of child survivors of Hurricane Andrew, 70% still manifested moderate to severe posttraumatic stress symptoms during a follow-up assessment conducted 21 months after the storm (Shaw et al. 1996). McFarlane (1987) found that 26 months after exposure to a bushfire in Australia, one-third of the children were still preoccupied with the disaster and continued to exhibit significant emotional and behavioral problems.

The Project Liberty counseling services utilization study (Covell et al. 2006) indicated that in the 27 months following the September 11 attacks, 9% of service recipients were children. The most common emotional reactions for children were sadness, tearfulness, anger and irritability, sleep disturbances, and intrusive thoughts and images. Younger children were more likely to experience anxiety, problems in concentration, social isolation, and withdrawal, whereas older children (ages 12–17) were more likely to exhibit numbing and avoidance reactions and to abuse substances. Fifteen months after Hurricane Katrina, Jaycox et al. (2010) found that 60% of New Orleans schoolchildren (in grades 4–8) screened positive for PTSD symptoms. McLaughlin et al. (2009) noted that 2 years after Hurricane Katrina 9.3% of 797 children ages 4–17 had a serious emotional disturbance directly attributable to the hurricane.

Studies of children exposed to child maltreatment, such as neglect and emotional, physical, or sexual abuse, have been found to have long-term changes in brain structure, including decreased brain volume (Cooper et al. 2007; De Bellis et al. 1999a, 1999b; Stover et al. 2007). Table 4–6 lists psychological responses to chronic trauma.

Common Stress Responses

Common stress responses that may occur with disaster exposure include anxiety symptoms, depressive and grief symptoms, behavioral symptoms, and somatic symptoms.

Anxiety symptoms.   Anxiety symptoms are present to varying degrees in virtually all persons exposed to trauma. These symptoms appear in multiple forms, such as fear and worries about recurrence; fears of dying or sustaining serious injury; worries about access to basic needs such as food, water, and safety and security; fears for loved ones and family members; and apprehension about the future.

Depressive and grief symptoms.   Depressive and grief symptoms frequently follow from the experiences of loss and change in the aftermath of disaster. These symptoms may appear as changes in mood and manifest as feelings of sadness, tearfulness, irritability, and hopelessness; loss of pleasure in previously enjoyed activities; decreased school performance; changes in interpersonal and social relationships; social avoidance, social withdrawal, and interpersonal conflicts; and changes in thinking such as decreased concentration, low self-esteem, diminished hope or preoccupation with suicide and death, and negative expectations about the future.

Behavioral symptoms.   Behavioral symptoms seen in persons exposed to trauma may include hyperactivity, agitation, belligerence, truancy from school, and deterioration in academic performance. Children or adolescents may initiate or increase engagement in unhealthy behaviors such as cigarette smoking, alcohol or drug use, or excessive use of prescription medications.

Somatic symptoms.   Somatic symptoms that might occur following disaster exposure include headaches, palpitations, appetite and sleep disturbance, difficulty breathing, gastrointestinal upset, and multiple unexplained physical symptoms.

Sleeper Effect

Some individuals may experience a delayed psychological response to an acute trauma. This so-called sleeper effect may occur when the maturing

TABLE 4–6.   Psychological responses to chronic trauma

Anxiety and mood disorders

Dissociation

Disruptive behaviors

Loss and grief reactions

Substance abuse

Personality changes

Suicidal behaviors

Psychiatric comorbidity

Somatic ills

Central nervous system changes

child acquires greater understanding of the consequences and ramifications of the traumatic experience that was not fully grasped at the time of the trauma. For example, a young girl who was sexually abused may have initially perceived the assault as an aggressive attack, but later she may fully understand the assault as sexual with all its ramifications.

Trauma-Specific Disorders

In some cases, the psychological responses to disaster are of sufficient magnitude to meet diagnostic criteria for a trauma-specific disorder such as acute stress disorder (ASD) or PTSD.

Acute Stress Disorder

ASD is diagnosed when an individual develops anxiety, dissociative, and related symptoms within 1 month after exposure to an extreme traumatic stressor (American Psychiatric Association 2000). This disturbance usually lasts for at least 2 days and does not persist beyond 4 weeks. Either while experiencing the traumatic event or after the event, the individual manifests at least three of the following dissociative symptoms: a subjective sense of numbing, detachment, or absence of emotional responsiveness; a reduction in awareness of his or her surroundings; derealization; depersonalization; or dissociative amnesia. Table 4–7 presents the DSM-IV-TR diagnostic criteria for ASD.

TABLE 4–7.   DSM-IV-TR diagnostic criteria for acute stress disorder

A. The person has been exposed to a traumatic event in which both of the following were present:

   (1) the person experienced, witnessed, or was confronted with an event or events that involved actual or threatened death or serious injury, or a threat to the physical integrity of self or others

   (2) the person's response involved intense fear, helplessness, or horror

B. Either while experiencing or after experiencing the distressing event, the individual has three (or more) of the following dissociative symptoms:

   (1) a subjective sense of numbing, detachment, or absence of emotional responsiveness

   (2) a reduction in awareness of his or her surroundings (e.g., "being in a daze")

   (3) derealization

   (4) depersonalization

   (5) dissociative amnesia (i.e., inability to recall an important aspect of the trauma)

C. The traumatic event is persistently reexperienced in at least one of the following ways: recurrent images, thoughts, dreams, illusions, flashback episodes, or a sense of reliving the experience; or distress on exposure to reminders of the traumatic event.

D. Marked avoidance of stimuli that arouse recollections of the trauma (e.g., thoughts, feelings, conversations, activities, places, people).

E. Marked symptoms of anxiety or increased arousal (e.g., difficulty sleeping, irritability, poor concentration, hypervigilance, exaggerated startle response, motor restlessness).

F. The disturbance causes clinically significant distress or impairment in social, occupational, or other important areas of functioning or impairs the individual's ability to pursue some necessary task, such as obtaining necessary assistance or mobilizing personal resources by telling family members about the traumatic experience.

G. The disturbance lasts for a minimum of 2 days and a maximum of 4 weeks and occurs within 4 weeks of the traumatic event.

H. The disturbance is not due to the direct physiological effects of a substance (e.g., a drug of abuse, a medication) or a general medical condition, is not better accounted for by brief psychotic disorder, and is not merely an exacerbation of a preexisting Axis I or Axis II disorder.

Source.   Reprinted from American Psychiatric Association 2000. Copyright 2000, American Psychiatric Association. Used with permission.

Dissociation symptoms, described briefly below, are important in the diagnosis of ASD:

- *Dissociation* describes the disconnection or lack of connection between things usually associated with each other (International Society for the Study of Trauma and Dissociation 2007). Usually the functions of consciousness, memory, identity, and perception are integrated and interconnected, but dissociation implies a separation among these functions. For example, a person experiencing emotional numbing may think about an event that was extremely upsetting yet have no feelings about it; in this case, thinking and feeling are disconnected.
- *Depersonalization* is the sense of being detached from and *not in* one's body; sometimes, this is described as an out-of-body experience.
- *Derealization* is the sense that the world is not real. Some persons have the sensation of watching the world as they would watch a movie.
- *Dissociative amnesia* refers to the inability to recall important personal information that goes well beyond ordinary forgetfulness. Disaster survivors may lack recall of major portions of the traumatic episode despite retaining consciousness during the disaster event.

ASD is characterized by a readiness to persistently reexperience intrusive images, dreams, thoughts, and perceptions associated with the disaster. The individual may consciously avoid any reminders that may arouse recollections of the trauma. To meet ASD clinical criteria, symptoms must cause clinically significant distress, interfere with normal functioning, or impair the individual's ability to meet the ordinary demands of everyday life. Finally, to qualify as ASD, the individual must experience at least one symptom from each of the three PTSD symptom clusters: 1) hyperarousal (difficulty sleeping, irritability, poor concentration, hypervigilance, exaggerated startle response, motor restlessness), 2) reexperiencing, and 3) avoidance.

Meiser-Stedman et al. (2007) studied 367 child survivors of motor vehicle crashes, ages 6–17 years, and found that only 9% met diagnostic criteria for ASD. However, another 18% met subsyndromal criteria because of the inability to fully document the dissociative symptoms. The authors concluded that the "excessively strict" dissociative criterion for youth makes ASD a rare diagnosis in children. Therefore, most children who do develop PTSD are not diagnosed with ASD in the month following trauma exposure (Stover et al. 2007).

Posttraumatic Stress Disorder

In 1980, the American Psychiatric Association introduced the diagnosis of PTSD into the psychiatric nomenclature. In contrast to other diagnoses, PTSD is noted to have a specific etiological agent in that "the person experienced, witnessed, or was confronted with an event or events that involved actual or threatened death or serious injury" usually associated with "fear, helplessness, or horror" (American Psychiatric Association 2000, p. 467). The diagnosis, with its clearly defined etiology, has been adopted with great enthusiasm. The DSM-IV-TR diagnostic criteria for PTSD are presented in Table 4–8.

Research focused on the psychological effects of trauma exposure—whether from natural disasters, such as hurricanes, floods, tsunamis, and earthquakes, or from human-generated disasters, such as acts of terrorism and aggressive assaults—has resulted in a plethora of reports documenting the existence of PTSD.

The lifetime prevalence of exposure to a traumatic event in which the individual is confronted with a real or imagined threat of physical injury or death is estimated at 70% for men and 50% for women (Kessler et al. 1995). Among those exposed to severe trauma, approximately 10% will meet threshold clinical criteria for PTSD, with twice as many women as men being so affected. Naturalistic studies indicate that men recover faster than women. Even 5 years following trauma, approximately one-third of adults with PTSD continue to meet diagnostic criteria (Breslau et al. 1998).

The compelling need of an individual with PTSD to relive, reexperience, and repeat the traumatic experience paradoxically oscillates with a need to avoid any thoughts, feelings, perceptions, or situations that remind him or her of the traumatic event (American Psychiatric Association 2000). Individuals are likely to vacillate between denial and a flooding of consciousness with intrusive images, thoughts, and perceptions, accompanied by their associated effects of fear, terror, and helplessness. PTSD diagnosis should be considered only for individuals whose symptoms persist for longer than 1 month.

A study of a representative sample of adults in Manhattan 5–8 weeks after the September 11 attack revealed that 19% reported a current history of PTSD, twice the rate of PTSD prior to the attack (Galea et al. 2002). Further, 58% of respondents reported at least one PTSD symptom. A diagnosis of PTSD was predicted by exposure to two or more stressors in the prior 12 months, a panic attack during or shortly after the attack, lack of social support, direct involvement in rescue efforts, and loss of personal possessions due to the event. The most common PTSD symptoms were intrusive memories (27%), insomnia (25%), and exaggerated startle reactions (24%).

TABLE 4–8.   DSM-IV-TR diagnostic criteria for posttraumatic stress disorder

---

A. The person has been exposed to a traumatic event in which both of the following were present:

   (1) the person experienced, witnessed, or was confronted with an event or events that involved actual or threatened death or serious injury, or a threat to the physical integrity of self or others

   (2) the person's response involved intense fear, helplessness, or horror.   **Note:** In children, this may be expressed instead by disorganized or agitated behavior

B. The traumatic event is persistently reexperienced in one (or more) of the following ways:

   (1) recurrent and intrusive distressing recollections of the event, including images, thoughts, or perceptions.   **Note:** In young children, repetitive play may occur in which themes or aspects of the trauma are expressed.

   (2) recurrent distressing dreams of the event.   **Note:** In children, there may be frightening dreams without recognizable content.

   (3) acting or feeling as if the traumatic event were recurring (includes a sense of reliving the experience, illusions, hallucinations, and dissociative flashback episodes, including those that occur on awakening or when intoxicated).   **Note:** In young children, trauma-specific reenactment may occur.

   (4) intense psychological distress at exposure to internal or external cues that symbolize or resemble an aspect of the traumatic event

   (5) physiological reactivity on exposure to internal or external cues that symbolize or resemble an aspect of the traumatic event

C. Persistent avoidance of stimuli associated with the trauma and numbing of general responsiveness (not present before the trauma), as indicated by three (or more) of the following:

   (1) efforts to avoid thoughts, feelings, or conversations associated with the trauma

   (2) efforts to avoid activities, places, or people that arouse recollections of the trauma

   (3) inability to recall an important aspect of the trauma

   (4) markedly diminished interest or participation in significant activities

---

TABLE 4–8. DSM-IV-TR diagnostic criteria for posttraumatic stress disorder *(continued)*

C. Persistent avoidance of stimuli associated with the trauma and numbing of general responsiveness *(continued):*

   (5) feeling of detachment or estrangement from others

   (6) restricted range of affect (e.g., unable to have loving feelings)

   (7) sense of a foreshortened future (e.g., does not expect to have a career, marriage, children, or a normal life span)

D. Persistent symptoms of increased arousal (not present before the trauma), as indicated by two (or more) of the following:

   (1) difficulty falling or staying asleep

   (2) irritability or outbursts of anger

   (3) difficulty concentrating

   (4) hypervigilance

   (5) exaggerated startle response

E. Duration of the disturbance (symptoms in Criteria B, C, and D) is more than 1 month.

F. The disturbance causes clinically significant distress or impairment in social, occupational, or other important areas of functioning.

Source. Reprinted from American Psychiatric Association: *Diagnostic and Statistical Manual of Mental Disorders,* 4th Edition, Text Revision. Washington, DC, American Psychiatric Association, 2000. Copyright 2000, American Psychiatric Association. Used with permission.

Various peritraumatic symptoms are known to predict future PTSD or other disaster-related psychopathology for both youth and adults. Prominent among these are panic, dissociation, feeling overwhelmed, and other extreme emotional responses (Flynn 2006; Lawyer et al. 2006). Stressors associated with disasters such as job loss, loss of property, death of loved ones, and displacement tend to exacerbate preexisting problems within families. In addition, maladaptive coping mechanisms such as increased substance abuse and increased domestic violence create hardships within families after a disaster.

Proposed Revision of Diagnostic Criteria for Posttraumatic Stress Disorder

Revisions to the DSM-IV (American Psychiatric Association 1994) PTSD criteria that are being considered for DSM-5 are listed in Table 4–9 (Friedman 2010). The following is a summary of the specific recommendations:

TABLE 4–9.	**Proposed revision for DSM-5 posttraumatic stress disorder**

A. The person was exposed to one or more of the following event(s): death or threatened death, actual or threatened serious injury, or actual or threatened sexual violation, in one or more of the following ways:

   (1) experiencing the event(s) him/herself

   (2) witnessing, in person, the event(s) as they occurred to others

   (3) learning that the event(s) occurred to a close relative or close friend; in such cases, the actual or threatened death must have been violent or accidental

   (4) experiencing repeated or extreme exposure to aversive details of the event(s) (e.g., first responders collecting body parts; police officers repeatedly exposed to details of child abuse); this does not apply to exposure through electronic media, television, movies, or pictures, unless this exposure is work related

B. Intrusion symptoms that are associated with the traumatic event(s) (that began after the traumatic event[s]), as evidenced by one or more of the following:

   (1) spontaneous or cued recurrent, involuntary, and intrusive distressing memories of the traumatic event(s).   **Note:** In children, repetitive play may occur in which themes or aspects of the traumatic event(s) are expressed.

   (2) recurrent distressing dreams in which the content and/or affect of the dream is related to the event(s).   **Note:** In children, there may be frightening dreams without recognizable content.

   (3) dissociative reactions (e.g., flashbacks) in which the individual feels or acts as if the traumatic event(s) were recurring. (Such reactions may occur on a continuum, with the most extreme expression being a complete loss of awareness of present surroundings.)   **Note:** In children, trauma-specific reenactment may occur in play.

   (4) intense or prolonged psychological distress at exposure to internal or external cues that symbolize or resemble an aspect of the traumatic event(s)

   (5) marked physiological reactions to reminders of the traumatic event(s)

TABLE 4–9. **Proposed revision for DSM-5 posttraumatic stress disorder** *(continued)*

C. Persistent avoidance of stimuli associated with the traumatic event(s) (that began after the traumatic event[s]), as evidenced by efforts to avoid one or more of the following:

  (1) internal reminders (thoughts, feelings, or physical sensations) that arouse recollections of the traumatic event(s)

  (2) external reminders (people, places, conversations, activities, objects, and situations) that arouse recollections of the traumatic event(s)

D. Negative alterations in cognitions and mood that are associated with the traumatic event(s) (that began or worsened after the traumatic event[s]), as evidenced by three or more of the following: **Note:** In children, as evidenced by two or more of the following:

  (1) inability to remember an important aspect of the traumatic event(s) (typically dissociative amnesia; not due to head injury, alcohol, or drugs)

  (2) persistent and exaggerated negative expectations about oneself, others, or the world (e.g., "I am bad," "No one can be trusted," "I've lost my soul forever," "My whole nervous system is permanently ruined," "The world is completely dangerous")

  (3) persistent distorted blame of self or others about the cause or consequences of the traumatic event(s)

  (4) pervasive negative emotional state (e.g., fear, horror, anger, guilt, or shame)

  (5) markedly diminished interest or participation in significant activities

  (6) feeling of detachment or estrangement from others

  (7) persistent inability to experience positive emotions (e.g., unable to have loving feelings, psychic numbing)

E. Alterations in arousal and reactivity that are associated with the traumatic event(s) (that began or worsened after the traumatic event[s]), as evidenced by three or more of the following: **Note:** In children, as evidenced by two or more of the following:

  (1) irritable or aggressive behavior

  (2) reckless or self-destructive behavior

  (3) hypervigilance

  (4) exaggerated startle response

  (5) problems with concentration

  (6) sleep disturbance (e.g., difficulty falling or staying asleep, restless sleep)

TABLE 4–9.   **Proposed revision for DSM-5 posttraumatic stress disorder** *(continued)*

F. Duration of the disturbance (symptoms in Criteria B, C, D, and E) is more than 1 month.

G. The disturbance causes clinically significant distress or impairment in social, occupational, or other important areas of functioning.

H. The disturbance is not due to the direct physiological effects of a substance (e.g., medication or alcohol) or a general medical condition (e.g., traumatic brain injury, coma).

Specify if:

With Delayed Onset: if diagnostic threshold is not exceeded until 6 months or more after the event(s) (although onset of some symptoms may occur sooner than this)

Source.   DSM-5 Development Web Site (http://www.dsm5.org/Proposed-Revision/Pages/proposedrevision.aspx?rid=165).

- DSM-IV Criterion A2, which requires an emotional response of "fear, helplessness, or horror" in response to a traumatic event, will be eliminated because the presence of such a response does not have clinical utility for predicting the onset of PTSD and the absence of such a response does not reduce the risk of PTSD.
- DSM-IV Criterion C, avoidance and numbing, will be divided into two symptom categories: Criterion C, avoidance symptoms, and Criterion D, negative cognitions and mood symptoms.
- New Criterion D will include dysphoric emotions such as fear, horror, shame, and anger, as well as negative attributions such as self-blame and negative expectations about the self and the future.
- DSM-IV Criterion D, persistent symptoms of increased arousal, will become Criterion E, which involves alterations in hyperarousal and reactivity. The criterion will be expanded to include irritable or aggressive behavior, and reckless and self-destructive behaviors, as well as sleep disturbance, hypervigilance, startle reactions, and concentration problems.

Proposed Revision of Diagnosis of Posttraumatic Stress Disorder in Preschool Children

Although considerable controversy exists regarding the diagnosis of PTSD in preschool children, there is general agreement that PTSD does occur in preschool children (Scheeringa 2008). An earlier study suggested that the prevalence rate of PTSD in traumatized preschool children is approximately 0.1%, considerably less than that reported for school-age children and adolescents, which is usually in the range of 3%–7% (Kirkpatrick et al. 2003; Scheeringa et al. 2003).

Several authors have suggested altering threshold criteria for the diagnosis of PTSD in preschool children such that symptoms are more developmentally sensitive. Scheeringa et al. (2003) suggested lowering the number of Criterion C items, related to numbing and avoidance, from three to one. In a later study, the authors indeed found that traumatized children under age 7 years rarely met the requirement for three Criterion C symptoms (Scheeringa et al. 2006). Meiser-Stedman et al. (2008), using parent report, evaluated children ages 2–6 years at 6 months following a motor vehicle accident using alternate criteria: 1) a decrease to one avoidance symptom and 2) removal of the requirement for Criterion A2, the experiencing of fear, helplessness, or horror at the time of the trauma. They found that 6.5% of the children met diagnostic criteria for PTSD based on the revised criteria compared with 1.6% based on DSM-IV criteria. Interestingly, when the authors evaluated children ages 7–10 years, they found no advantage for the alternate criteria over the DSM-IV criteria when both parent and child report were included. Proposed DSM-5 revisions for PTSD criteria in preschool children are listed in Table 4–10.

Posttraumatic Stress Disorder in Children and Adolescents After Disaster

There is increasing recognition of the importance of identification of PTSD in children and adolescents (Cohen et al. 2010). Copeland et al. (2007) found that two-thirds of children in the Great Smoky Mountain Study reported having experienced at least one traumatic event before age 16 and that 14% had experienced one or more posttraumatic stress symptoms. Giaconia et al. (1995), in a longitudinal study of a community-based sample of 384 adolescents, found that 40% had experienced at least one traumatic event by age 18 and that 14.5% of this group had developed PTSD.

The baseline rate of PTSD is estimated to range from 3% to 6% in school-age children (Reinherz et al. 1993; Scheeringa et al. 2003). In a national survey of adolescents ages 13–17, Kilpatrick et al. (2003) indicated that 3.7% of males and 6.3% of females met diagnostic criteria for PTSD.

Following the September 11 attack, a survey of 8,266 New York City children in grades 4–12 indicated that the rate of PTSD increased from 2% to 10% and the rate of separation anxiety disorder doubled (Fremont 2004). Children who developed PTSD and other less severe psycholog-

---

TABLE 4–10. Proposed DSM-5 revision for posttraumatic stress disorder in preschool children

---

A. The child (less than 6 years old) was exposed to the following event(s): death or threatened death, actual or threatened serious injury, or actual or threatened sexual violation, in one or more of the following ways:

   (1) experiencing the event(s) him/herself

   (2) witnessing the event(s) as it (they) occurred to others, especially primary caregivers

   (3) learning that the event(s) occurred to a close relative or close friend* **Note:** Witnessing does not include event(s) that are witnessed only in electronic media, television, movies, or pictures.

B. Intrusion symptoms that are associated with the traumatic event(s) (that began after the traumatic event[s]), as evidenced by one or more of the following:

   (1) spontaneous or cued recurrent, involuntary, and intrusive distressing memories of the traumatic event(s).
   Note: Spontaneous and intrusive memories may not necessarily appear distressing and may be expressed as play reenactment.

   (2) recurrent distressing dreams related to the traumatic event(s). **Note:** It may not be possible to ascertain that the content is related to the traumatic event(s).

   (3) dissociative reactions in which the individual feels or acts as if the traumatic event(s) were recurring (such reactions may occur on a continuum with the most extreme expression being a complete loss of awareness of present surroundings)

   (4) intense or prolonged psychological distress at exposure to internal or external cues that symbolize or resemble an aspect of the traumatic event(s)

   (5) marked physiological reactions to reminders of the traumatic event(s)

One item from C or D below:

C. Persistent avoidance of stimuli associated with the traumatic event (that began after the traumatic event), as evidenced by efforts to avoid:

   (1) activities, places, or physical reminders that arouse recollections of the traumatic event

   (2) people, conversations, or interpersonal situations that arouse recollections of the traumatic event

TABLE 4–10. Proposed DSM-5 revision for posttraumatic stress disorder in preschool children (*continued*)

D. Negative alterations in cognitions and mood that are associated with the traumatic event (that began or worsened after the traumatic event), as evidenced by one or more of the following:

  (1) substantially increased frequency of negative emotional states (e.g., fear, guilt, sadness, shame, or confusion)*

  (2) markedly diminished interest or participation in significant activities, including constriction of play

  (3) socially withdrawn behavior

  (4) persistent reduction in expression of positive emotions

E. Alterations in arousal and reactivity that are associated with the traumatic event (that began or worsened after the traumatic event), as evidenced by two or more of the following:

  (1) irritable, angry, or aggressive behavior, including extreme temper tantrums

  (2) reckless or self-destructive behavior*

  (3) hypervigilance

  (4) exaggerated startle response

  (5) problems with concentration

  (6) sleep disturbance (e.g., difficulty falling or staying asleep, restless sleep)

F. Duration of the disturbance (symptoms in Criteria B, C, D, and E) is more than 1 month.

G. The disturbance causes clinically significant distress or impairment in relationships with parents, siblings, peers, or other caregivers, or in school behavior.

*At present, there is not a consensus about including these items. Data relevant to their inclusion or exclusion are being sought.
Source. DSM-5 Development Web Site (http://www.dsm5.org/Proposed-Revision/Pages/proposedrevision.aspx?rid=396).

ical responses continued to manifest ongoing psychological difficulties long after the terrorist event. Research suggests that 30%–50% of the children exposed to a terrorist act experience one or more of the following: PTSD, anxiety disorders, somatic ills, mood disorders, and disturbances in development and behavior.

 Disaster exposure is increasingly being found to be associated with long-term mental health effects. Two years after the 1972 Buffalo Creek disaster, a flood caused by the failure of a coal slurry impoundment dam, 30% of children younger than 8 years and 39% of children older than 8 years met criteria for PTSD (Green et al. 1991). A 14-year follow-up of the Buffalo Creek child survivors revealed that 28% still had PTSD (Green et al. 1990). Even 17 years after the event, 7% of the children, all females, still met diagnostic criteria for PTSD (Green et al. 1994).

A prospective longitudinal study of 2,548 German adolescents and young adults, ages 14–24, who had been exposed to either assaultive behavior or serious accidents found that 125 (5%) met DSM-IV criteria for PTSD (20%) or subthreshold PTSD (80%) at baseline (Perkonigg et al. 2005). Over half of those with PTSD remained symptomatic for more than 3 years, and 43% of those with subthreshold PTSD continued to be significantly symptomatic or to meet diagnostic criteria for PTSD.

Complex Trauma

Complex trauma refers to repeated exposure to violence that begins in childhood and is continued throughout the developmental years. The accumulation of traumatic episodes occurring in childhood, frequently characteristic of child maltreatment, war-related trauma, and other repeated exposures, is associated with a more complex psychological presentation than can be explained by PTSD and extends beyond symptoms of reexperiencing, avoidance, and hyperarousal. The psychological responses to repetitive traumatic events can best be conceptualized as a trauma syndrome or as a disorder of extreme stress in which those responses to the trauma become woven into the fabric of personality, with mood and affective dysregulation, identity conflicts, altered self-attributions, damaged self-efficacy, altered interpersonal relationships, inattention, and altered systems of meaning, as well as somatic symptoms (Pelcovitz et al. 1997; Roth et al. 1997).

An example of an individual with complex trauma is a child soldier from the Congo, who reported a history of laughing uncontrollably and being filled with anger and that killing had become as easy as drinking water, and indicated that he was unable to think. He said he was so sad that his "bones started to ache" (Beah 2007, p. 72). He complained that his emotions were in disarray and that he could not comprehend what or how he felt. He felt that nobody could be trusted and that everybody was after him, and lamented that his innocence had been replaced by fear and that he had become a monster. He craved cocaine and marijuana.

Other Psychiatric Disorders Often Associated With Disaster

Because of the well-described PTSD threshold criteria and the specific descriptions of symptoms, trauma and PTSD are often considered as being virtually synonymous, as if trauma always leads to PTSD. Too often, diagnostic instruments that address only PTSD are used instead of those that assess a wider spectrum of psychological responses to trauma exposure. Although the diagnosis of PTSD has been a wonderful focus for research, it has been somewhat of a confound when a clinician has to respond to the psychological needs of those exposed to trauma. The diagnosis has all too frequently limited the attention and therapeutic focus of clinicians, who instead need to be sensitive to the complexity and diversity of the psychological responses to trauma as they occur across a timeline that is frequently mediated by a host of secondary stressors. Many clinicians have come to think of the psychological responses to trauma as totally within the conceptual understanding of PTSD.

Usually, a child or adolescent who meets the diagnostic criteria for PTSD will manifest other psychological and psychiatric problems. Giaconia et al. (1995) found that 80% of older adolescents with a diagnosis of PTSD met criteria for an additional psychiatric diagnosis and 40% met criteria for two or more other psychiatric diagnoses, usually anxiety and mood disorders.

In the Great Smoky Mountain Study, Copeland et al. (2007) found that although two-thirds of the children had been exposed to a traumatic event by age 16, a diagnosis of PTSD was rare across middle childhood and adolescence. Only 0.5% met the diagnostic criteria for PTSD, whereas 13.4% developed some posttraumatic stress symptoms. Children who had been exposed to trauma had double the rates of psychiatric diagnoses of those not exposed, suggesting the widening spectrum of psychological responses to trauma.

Exposure to an increasing number of traumatic events results in a cumulative effect, putting children at increased risk for anxiety, depressive behavioral diagnoses, and substance abuse.

Anxiety Disorders

Commonly coexisting with PTSD are anxiety disorders such as separation anxiety disorder, generalized anxiety disorder, and specific phobias. In a recent study, Merikangas et al. (2011) documented that only

36.2% of adolescents receive mental health services for mental disorders, and only 17.8% of adolescents with an anxiety disorder receive services because most services are directed toward those with more manifest behavioral problems.

Mood Disorders

Depressive symptoms occur in 10%–40% of individuals exposed to trauma. The most common coexisting mood disorders are major depression and dysthymia (chronically depressed mood lasting longer than 1 year). Approximately 75% of adults with PTSD have coexisting psychiatric diagnoses, with 35%–45% having a lifetime history of depression (Breslau et al. 1998). Giaconia et al. (1995) found that 43% of older adolescents with PTSD also met criteria for a major depressive disorder. The PTSD preceded or occurred at the same age as major depression for 70% of the adolescents. Kar and Bastia (2006) noted that 18% of adolescents manifested a major mood disorder following exposure to a cyclone. In a longitudinal study of adult primary care patient survivors of the September 11 attack, Neria et al. (2010) found that a diagnosis of major depressive disorder before the attack was the strongest predictor of PTSD and late-onset PTSD, 1 and 4 years, respectively, after exposure to the event.

Mood symptoms in children are comparable to those experienced by adults, with some exceptions. For example, younger children frequently display somatic symptoms and regressive clinging and dependent behaviors, whereas adolescents are more likely to engage in suicidal thoughts or actions and to increase substance abuse behaviors. Symptoms of depression are listed in Table 4–11.

Behavior Disorders

Children (primarily boys) exposed to traumatic events may demonstrate disturbances in behavior such as attention-deficit/hyperactivity disorder, oppositional defiant disorder, conduct disorder, substance abuse, and various physical complaints. Giaconia et al. (1995) found a significant correlation between PTSD and externalizing behaviors (behavioral problems) in older adolescents. Shaw et al. (1995) found a temporary decrease in school-based disruptive behaviors immediately after Hurricane Andrew but noted an increase in such behaviors over the next 21 months.

TABLE 4–11. Symptoms of depression

Changes in mood	Feelings of sadness and depression
	Irritability
	Loss of interest in pleasurable activities
Changes in behavior	Changes in personality
	Changes in school performance
	Loss of interest in previously enjoyed activities
	Tearfulness
	Impaired functioning
Changes in relationship	Social avoidance
	Social withdrawal or isolation
	Interpersonal conflicts
	Family conflicts
Changes in thinking	Low self-esteem
	Self-deprecation
	Self-absorption
	Feelings of hopelessness and helplessness
	Demoralization
	Inability to think or concentrate
	Preoccupation with death or suicide
	Negative expectations about the future
Changes in bodily functioning	Change in appetite and body weight
	Change in sleep pattern
	Change in activity level
	Somatic complaints

Substance Abuse and Adolescents

The relationship between trauma and substance abuse is an area of investigation that is slowly evolving. Paradoxically, trauma is a risk factor for substance abuse, and substance abuse is a risk factor for trauma exposure. Although adolescents are usually strong and healthy, rates of injury and death will increase by 200% from childhood to adulthood (Institute of Medicine and National Research Council [IOM and NRC] 2011). Adolescents are more likely to engage in reckless behavior and not infrequently put their health and sometimes even their lives in danger. Although impulsivity decreases between ages 10 and 30 years, sensation-seeking behaviors increase between ages 10 and 15 years (IOM and NRC 2011). All too frequently, adolescents engage in unsafe driving, unsafe sex, and youth violence; have a readiness to experiment with illegal drugs, alcohol, and tobacco; and are more likely to engage in delinquent activities. Seventy percent of all deaths in the second decade of life are caused by motor vehicle accidents, suicide, or homicide (IOM and NRC 2011).

The IOM and NRC (2011) report provides some startling statistics for 2005: one in three deaths of teenagers was related to a motor vehicle accident; 3.4 million teenagers annually were victims of violence; and one-third of all firearm deaths among teenagers were self-inflicted. Also, 17% of youth contemplated suicide, and 13% said they had made a suicide plan. The increase in adolescent risk-taking behavior is thought to be related to marked changes in brain structure.

During puberty, pruning of synaptic connections occurs: an estimated 30,000 synapses are lost every second, and synaptic connections decrease by approximately 50% (Spear 2007). Pruning seems to be more pronounced in the prefrontal cortex, with an overall decrease in gray matter and an increase in white matter throughout the brain. Spear (2007) suggested that alterations in the dopaminergic system during puberty may lead to a "mild or partial anhedonia," which may result in the adolescents' seeking of environmental novelty, drugs, and other sensations as a behavioral remediation for a reward deficiency. She suggested that "exaggerated sensitivity to the rewards offered by many high-risk behaviors, and a reduced sensitivity to adverse effects and the insufficient power of immature frontal cognitive controls all contribute to adolescent risk taking" (Spear 2007, p. 20).

The misuse of substances (i.e., drugs of abuse, medications, or toxins; American Psychiatric Association 2000) increases across the teenage years, with different levels of severity and individual risk. As teenagers progress through high school, their use of tobacco doubles; alcohol use increases from 38.9% to 72.2%; marijuana use increases from 14.2% to 41.8%; and their use of illegal substances other than marijuana increases from 11.1% to 25.5%%. Variations occur in the amount imbibed, the frequency and dose, and the levels of impairment. In contrast to adults, adolescents are at higher risk for bingeing behavior as part of their experimentation. Boys are more likely to use substances, and poverty has been found to be a risk factor for increased use of substances (IOM and NRC 2011). Dual diagnosis is common with other psychiatric disorders.

A clinician needs to distinguish between patterns of substance misuse. *Substance use* refers to consumption of illicit drugs, which for underage youth include alcohol. A range of medications may be abused, from over-the-counter medications to a host of prescription medications. A continuum of behaviors exists, ranging from experimentation, to recreational use, to a pattern of use associated with various levels of impairment.

DSM-IV-TR (American Psychiatric Association 2000) distinguishes between substance abuse disorder and substance dependence. *Substance abuse disorder* refers to recurrent use of a substance, leading to a pattern of maladaptive behavior that results in significant impairment or distress often associated with failure to fulfill obligations at work, school, or home. Frequently, this disorder is associated with legal, interpersonal, and social problems and behaviors, such as unsafe driving, that lead to increased risk of injury. *Substance dependence* is a disorder associated with evidence of impairment and/or distress and is characterized by a 12-month period of recurrent drug use leading to increasing tolerance — that is, a need for increased amounts to achieve the same level of desired effect — and symptoms of withdrawal when the substance is no longer available. In a recent utilization study, Merikangas et al. (2011) documented that only 15.4% of adolescents with a substance abuse disorder receive specific treatment services for their condition.

An estimated 33%–59% of women and 12%–34% of men in substance abuse treatment have a concurrent diagnosis of PTSD (Najavits 2002). Kessler et al. (1995), in a survey of a community sample, found that 52% of male subjects with PTSD were also diagnosed with alcohol abuse or dependence, compared with 34% of those without PTSD. Women were more likely to have experienced sexual or physical abuse, whereas men were more likely to have been exposed to violent crime or war-related trauma. Triffleman et al. (1995) found that 40% of substance-abusing veterans in an inpatient setting had a history of combat PTSD, and 38% had a current diagnosis of PTSD. Individuals with dual diagnoses are more likely to abuse hard drugs, such as cocaine and heroin, as well as more established drugs, such as alcohol and marijuana, in an attempt to self-medicate posttraumatic stress symptoms, and they are more likely to have been exposed to repeated trauma (Najavits 2002).

Little systematic research exists on the relationship between exposure to natural disaster and adolescent substance abuse. Schroeder and Polusny (2004) found that adolescents experiencing posttraumatic stress symptoms after exposure to a tornado were at an increased risk for alcohol use. In a study of 280 adolescents exposed to Hurricane Rita, Rohrbach et al. (2009) found a positive correlation between posttraumatic stress symptoms and the use of alcohol and marijuana at 7 months after exposure.

A survey of 297 adolescents ages 15–19 in a treatment program for substance abuse found that the lifetime prevalence of PTSD was 30%, five times greater than that reported for a community-based sample (Deykin and Buka 1997). Giaconia et al. (1995, 2000), in a study of 384 adolescents, reported that an association existed between PTSD in adolescents and substance dependence and that for most adolescents (45%–66%) the substance abuse disorder preceded the onset of trauma exposure (Giaconia et al. 2000). Thirty-three percent had a substance use disorder, 43% had had trauma exposure, and 18.5% had coexisting substance use disorder and trauma exposure. The authors found that in half the cases of alcohol use, the use of alcohol increased the risk of PTSD, and half the time the PTSD preceded the onset of alcohol use, confirming that alcohol use is often associated with a higher risk of injury. Adolescents with a history of excessive alcohol use are 6–12 times more likely to have a history of trauma exposure (Clark et al. 1997).

Resilience

Resilience is a measure of an individual's capacity to rapidly restore predisaster levels of function and psychological equilibrium. According to Henderson Grotberg (2001), resilience involves the capacity to cope with and be strengthened or transformed by adversity experiences, such as disasters. Rutter (1987) noted that children with good coping skills, self-mastery, easy temperament, and a history of a good relationship with an adult were more resistant and less vulnerable to psychopathology in later life. Garmezy et al. (1984) and Werner and Smith (1982) stressed the importance of early family relationships, self-efficacy, and an inner conviction that one's life is within one's control as factors contributing to resilience. Factors that enhance child resilience are effective parenting, positive self-concept, self-regulation, social competence, cognitive flexibility, adaptability to new situations, problem-solving skills, ease with transitions, communication skills, empathy, assertiveness in one's self-interest, humor, religious affiliation, and the ability to elicit caretaking behaviors (Masten 2007).

Masten (2007) emphasized that early attachments and healthy caregiver relationships that provide emotional security facilitate prosocial behaviors, tolerance for frustration, effective information processing, self-regulation, stress management, and adaptability. She acknowledged the important influences of the school and community in fostering the child's socialization and providing opportunities for mastery and learning. Integral to resilience are the child's accrued "competencies," including elements of academic, social, interpersonal, and phase-specific mastery (Masten 2007). Genetics, neurotransmitters, and stress response systems have an important role in resilience. Some individuals appear to release higher levels of neuropeptide Y and allopregnanolone (a product of the adrenal glands) in response to stress; these reactions appear to confer natural resilience and to diminish anxiety (Hoge et al. 2007). In contrast, children who sustain prolonged exposure to poor parenting and nurturance may experience detrimental neurobiological and neurohormonal changes (e.g., decreased levels of oxytocin, a neurohormone believed to facilitate emotional bonding to others), thereby compromising social relatedness (Cooper et al. 2007; Hoge et al. 2007). Conversely, evidence indicates that a short form of the serotonin transporter gene may be associated with decreased resilience and increased risk for depression (Gunnar 2007). Table 4–12 lists factors that enhance resilience in children and adolescents.

Posttraumatic Growth

Traumatic events to which children may be exposed as part of their life experience include natural disasters, physical or sexual abuse, community violence, motor vehicle accidents, and so forth. Increasing awareness of the frequency of these experiences has led to an emerging interest in possible positive growth-promoting changes that may occur secondary to trauma exposure. *Posttraumatic growth* has been defined as a significant improvement in cognitive and emotional life that may have behavioral implications (Salter and Stallard 2004). Adult studies have confirmed that trauma may lead to positive effects, such as a greater sense of self-reliance and personal strength (Calhoun and Tedeschi 2004). Unfortunately, few studies have been done with children.

In a study of 46 children, ages 6–15 years, who had been exposed to Hurricane Floyd, Cryder et al. (2006) found that children subsequently often experienced an increasing sense of competence, particularly in a supportive social environment. A study of children, ages 7–10 years, after Hurricane Katrina found that although few of the children spontaneously expressed positive changes, there was some suggestion of increased spirituality, which was thought to reflect the parental and regional cultural value set placed on religion (Kilmer et al. 2009). A study of 158 children, ages 7–17 years, who had been involved in motor vehicle accidents found that 42% reported some posttraumatic growth, such as improved interpersonal relationships and a greater appreciation of life experiences (Salter and Stallard 2004). Interestingly, 37% of those who reported personal

TABLE 4–12.	**Factors that enhance resilience in children and adolescents**

Individual protective factors

Capacity to recognize opportunities in adversity

Problem-solving and emotional coping skills

Good social skills with peers and adults

Personal awareness of strengths and limitations

Feelings of empathy for others

Internal locus of control — a belief that one's efforts can make a difference

Sense of humor

Positive self-concept

Self-reliance

Cognitive flexibility

Positive emotions (optimism, sense of humor, interests, joy)

Ability to interact positively with others

Active coping

Physical exercise

Religion

Family protective factors

Positive family ambience

Good parent-child relationships

Parental harmony

A valued social role in the household, such as helping siblings or doing household chores

Community protective factors

Strong social support networks

Supportive extended family

A close relationship with unrelated mentor

Good peer relationships

Community influences that offer positive role models

Positive school experiences

Valued social role such as a job, volunteering, or helping neighbors

Membership in a religious or faith community

Extracurricular activities

Source. Cooper et al. 2007; Newman and Blackburn 2002.

growth also met criteria for PTSD, suggesting a possible topic of research. These findings were substantiated by Alisic et al. (2008), who surveyed children ages 8–12 who had been exposed to a traumatic event (DSM-IV Criterion A1) and found that posttraumatic stress reactions were positively correlated with posttraumatic growth. Among the factors that appear to mediate the potential for positive posttraumatic growth are family and social supports, previous trauma exposure, resilience, and the cascade of secondary stressors often associated with trauma exposure.

■ Key Clinical Points

- ■ Depending on the nature of the trauma, children may experience posttraumatic stress symptoms, anxiety symptoms, grief, depression, and somatic or behavioral responses.

- ■ Acute stress reactions are experienced by the majority of children exposed to disaster and are often manifested by distress and fears of recurrence.

- ■ Chronic stress reactions may occur in children who are particularly vulnerable or in those who are subjected to a cascade of postdisaster adversities.

- ■ For some children, psychological responses to disaster are sufficiently severe and distressing to meet criteria for trauma-specific disorders, such as acute stress disorder or posttraumatic stress disorder.

- ■ Posttraumatic stress disorder rarely occurs in isolation, and one should always look for coexisting psychological morbidities.

- ■ Adolescence is recognized as a period of increased trauma exposure. Adolescents are more likely to engage in reckless behavior and are at risk for substance abuse behaviors.

- ■ *Resilience* is mastery against adversity, and most children exhibit this capacity to overcome the challenges posed by disaster, restore equilibrium, and even emerge stronger and exhibit posttraumatic growth.

References

Alisic E, van der Schoot, van Ginkel JR, et al: Looking beyond posttraumatic stress disorder in children: posttraumatic stress reactions, posttraumatic growth and quality of life in a general population sample. J Clin Psychiatry 69:1455–1461, 2008

American Psychiatric Association: Diagnostic and Statistical Manual of Mental Disorders, 3rd Edition. Washington, DC, American Psychiatric Association, 1980

American Psychiatric Association: Diagnostic and Statistical Manual of Mental Disorders, 4th Edition. Washington, DC, American Psychiatric Association, 1994

American Psychiatric Association: Diagnostic and Statistical Manual of Mental Disorders, 4th Edition, Text Revision. Washington, DC, American Psychiatric Association, 2000

Bloch D, Silber E, Perry S: Some factors in the emotional reactions of children to disaster. Am J Psychiatry 113:416–422, 1956

Beah I: A Long Way Gone: Memoirs of a Boy Soldier. New York, Farrar, Straus, & Giroux, 2007

Breslau N, Kessler RC, Chilcoat HD, et al: Trauma and posttraumatic stress disorder in the community: the 1996 Detroit Area Survey of Trauma. Arch Gen Psychiatry 55:626–632, 1998

Calhoun LG, Tedeschi RG: The foundations of posttraumatic growth: new considerations. Psychological Inquiry 15:93–102, 2004

Clark DB, Lesnick L, Hegedus AM: Traumas and other adverse life events in adolescents with alcohol abuse and dependence. J Am Acad Child Adolesc Psychiatry 36:1744–1751, 1997

Cohen JA, Bukstein O, Walter H, et al; AACAP Work Group on Quality Issues: Practice parameter for the assessment and treatment of children and adolescents with posttraumatic stress disorder. J Am Acad Child Adolesc Psychiatry 49:414–431, 2010

Cooper NS, Feder A, Southwick AM, et al: Resiliency and vulnerability to trauma, in Adolescent Psychopathology and the Developing Brain. Edited by Romer D, Walker EF. Oxford, UK, Oxford University Press, 2007

Copeland WE, Keeler G, Angold A, et al: Traumatic events and posttraumatic stress in childhood. Arch Gen Psychiatry 64:577–584, 2007

Covell NH, Allen G, Foster MJ, et al: Service utilization and event reaction patterns among children who received Project Liberty counseling. Psychiatr Serv 57:1277–1282, 2006

Cryder CH, Kilmer RP, Tedeschi RG, et al: An exploratory study of posttraumatic growth in children following a natural disaster. Am J Orthopsychiatry 76:65–69, 2006

De Bellis MD, Baum AS, Birmaher B, et al: A.E. Bennett Research Award. Developmental traumatology, part I: biological stress systems. Biol Psychiatry 45:1259–1270, 1999a

De Bellis MD, Keshavan MS, Clark DB, et al: A.E. Bennett Research Award. Developmental traumatology, part II: brain development. Biol Psychiatry 45:1271–1284, 1999b

Deykin EY, Buka SL: Prevalence and risk factors for posttraumatic stress disorder among chemically dependent adolescents. Am J Psychiatry 154:752–757, 1997

Flynn BW: Meeting the needs of special populations in disaster and emergencies: making it work in rural areas. Presentation at the National Association for Rural Health, San Antonio, TX, August 22, 2006

Fremont W: Childhood reactions to terrorism-induced trauma: a review of the past 10 years. J Am Acad Child Adolesc Psychiatry 43:381–392, 2004

Friedman MJ: PTSD revisions proposed for DSM-5, with input from array of experts. Psychiatric News, May 21, 2010, p. 8. Available at: http://pn.psychiatryonline.org/content/45/10/8.full. Accessed August 24, 2011.

Galea S, Resnick H, Ahern J, et al: Posttraumatic stress disorder in Manhattan, New York City, after the September 11th terrorist attacks. J Urban Health 79:340–353, 2002

Garmezy N, Masten A, Tellegen A: The study of stress and competence in children: a building block for developmental psychopathology. Child Dev 55:97–111, 1984

Giaconia RM, Reinherz HZ, Silverman AB, et al: Trauma and posttraumatic stress disorder in a community population of older adolescents. J Am Acad Child Adolesc Psychiatry 34:1369–1380, 1995

Giaconia RM, Reinherz HZ, Hauf AC, et al: Comorbidity of substance use and posttraumatic stress disorders in a community sample of adolescents. Am J Orthopsychiatry 70:253–262, 2000

Green BL, Lindy JD, Grace MC, et al: Buffalo Creek survivors in the second decade: stability of stress symptoms. Am J Orthopsychiatry 60:43–54, 1990

Green BL, Korol M, Grace MC, et al: Children and disaster: age, gender and parental effects on PTSD symptoms. J Am Acad Child Adolesc Psychiatry 30:945–951, 1991

Green BL, Grace MC, Vary MG, et al: Children of disaster in the second decade: a 17-year follow-up of Buffalo Creek survivors. J Am Acad Child Adolesc Psychiatry 33:71–79, 1994

Gunnar MR: Stress effects on the developing brain, in Adolescent Psychopathology and the Developing Brain. Edited by Romer D, Walker EF. Oxford, UK, Oxford University Press, 2007, pp 127–147

Henderson Grotberg E: Resilience programs for children in disaster. Ambulatory Child Health 7:75–83, 2001

Hoge EA, Austin ED, Pollack MH: Resilience: research evidence and conceptual considerations for posttraumatic stress disorder. Depress Anxiety 24:139–152, 2007

Hoven CW, Durate CS, Turner JB, et al: Child mental health in the aftermath of disaster: a review of PTSD studies, in Mental Health and Disaster. Edited by Neria Y, Galea S, Norris FH. Cambridge, UK, Cambridge University Press 2009, pp 218–232

Institute of Medicine: Preparing for the Psychological Consequences of Terrorism: A Public Health Strategy. Washington, DC, National Academies Press, 2003

Institute of Medicine and National Research Council Committee on the Science of Adolescence: The Science of Adolescent Risk-Taking: Workshop Report. Washington, DC, National Academies Press, 2011

International Society for the Study of Trauma and Dissociation: Frequently Asked Questions: Dissociation and Dissociative Disorders. 2007. Available at: www.isst-d.org/education/faq-dissociation.htm. Accessed August 24, 2011.

Jaycox LH, Cohen JA, Manarino AP, et al: Children's mental health care following Hurricane Katrina: a field trial of trauma-focused psychotherapies. J Trauma Stress 23:223–231, 2010

Kar N, Bastia BK: Post-traumatic stress disorder, depression and generalized anxiety disorder in adolescents after a natural disaster: a study of comorbidity. Clin Pract Epidemiol Ment Health 2:17, 2006

Kessler RC, Sonnega A, Bromet E, et al: Posttraumatic stress disorder in the National Comorbidity Survey. Arch Gen Psychiatry 52:1048–1060, 1995

Kilmer RP, Gil-Rivas V, Tedeschi RG, et al: Use of the Posttraumatic Growth Inventory for Children. J Trauma Stress 22:248–253, 2009

Kilpatrick DG, Ruggiero KJ, Acierno R, et al: Violence and risk of PTSD, major depression, substance abuse/dependence, and comorbidity: results from the National Survey of Adolescents. J Consult Clin Psychology 71:692–700, 2003

Lawyer SR, Resnick HS, Galea S, et al: Predictors of peritraumatic reactions of PTSD following the September 11th terrorist attacks. Psychiatry 69:130–141, 2006

Masten A: Competence, resilience and development, in Adolescent Psychopathology and the Developing Brain. Edited by Romer D, Walker EF. Oxford, UK, Oxford University Press, 2007, pp 31–52

McFarlane AC: Posttraumatic phenomena in a longitudinal study of children following a natural disaster. J Am Acad Child Adolesc Psychiatry 26:764–769, 1987

McLaughlin KA, Fairbanks JA, Gruber MJ, et al: Serious emotional disturbance among youths exposed to Hurricane Katrina 2 years postdisaster. J Am Acad Child Adolesc Psychiatry 48:1069–1078, 2009

Meiser-Stedman R, Dalgleish T, Smith P, et al: Dissociative symptoms and the acute stress disorder diagnosis in children and adolescents: a replication of the Harvey and Bryant (1999) study. J Trauma Stress 20:359–364, 2007

Meiser-Stedman R, Smith P, Gluckman E, et al: The posttraumatic stress disorder diagnosis in preschool- and elementary school-age children exposed to motor vehicle accidents. Am J Psychiatry 165:1326–1337, 2008

Merikangas KR, He J, Burstein M, et al: Service utilization for lifetime mental disorders in U.S. adolescents: results of the National Comorbidity Survey, Adolescent Supplement. J Am Acad Child Adolesc Psychiatry 50:32–45, 2011

Najavits L: Seeking Safety: A Treatment Manual for PTSD and Substance Abuse. New York, Guilford Press, 2002

National Child Traumatic Stress Network: Child Welfare Trauma Training Toolkit. Los Angeles,, CA, National Child Traumatic Stress Network, 2008

National Commission on Children and Disasters: 2010 Report to the President and Congress (AHRQ Publ No 10-M037). Rockville, MD, Agency for Healthcare Research and Quality, October 2010. Available at: http://www.acf.hhs.gov/ohsepr/nccdreport. Accessed August 25, 2011.

Neria Y, Olfson M, DiGrande L, et al: Long-term course of probable PTSD after 9/11 attacks: a study in urban primary care. J Trauma Stress 23:474–482, 2010

Neuner F, Schauer E, Catani C, et al: Post-tsunami stress: a study of posttraumatic stress disorder in children living in three severely affected regions in Sri Lanka. J Trauma Stress 19:339–347, 2006

Newman T, Blackburn S: Transitions in the Lives of Children and Young People: Resilience Factors. October 25, 2002. Available at: http://www.scotland.gov.uk/Publications/2002/10/15591/11950. Accessed August 24, 2011.

Pelcovitz D, van der Kolk B, Roth S, et al: Development of a criteria set and a structured interview for disorders of extreme stress (SIDES). J Trauma Stress 10:3–16, 1997

Perkonigg A, Pfister H, Stein MB, et al: Longitudinal course of posttraumatic stress disorder and posttraumatic stress disorder symptoms in a community sample of adolescents and young adults. Am J Psychiatry 162:1320–1327, 2005

Piaget J: Six Psychological Studies. New York, Random House, 1967

Pynoos RS, Nader K: Psychological first aid and treatment approach to children exposed to community violence. J Trauma Stress 1:445–473, 1988

Reinherz HZ, Giaconia RM, Lefkowitz ES, et al: Prevalence of psychiatric disorders in a community population of older adolescents. J Am Acad Child Adolesc Psychiatry 32:369–377, 1993

Rohrbach LA, Grana R, Vernberg E, et al: Impact of Hurricane Rita on adolescent substance abuse. Psychiatry 72:222–237, 2009

Roth S, Newman E, Pelcovitz D, et al: Complex PTSD in victims exposed to sexual and physical abuse: results from the DSM-IV field trial for posttraumatic stress disorder. J Trauma Stress 10:539–555, 1997

Rutter M: Psychosocial resilience and protective mechanisms. Am J Orthopsychiatry 57:316–331, 1987

Salter E, Stallard P: Posttraumatic growth in child survivors of a road traffic accident. J Trauma Stress 17:335–340, 2004

Scheeringa MS: Developmental considerations for diagnosing PTSD and acute stress disorder in preschool and school-age children. Am J Psychiatry 165:1237–1239, 2008

Scheeringa M, Zeanah C, Myers L, et al: New findings on alternative criteria for PTSD in preschool children. J Am Acad Child Adolesc Psychiatry 42:561–570, 2003

Scheeringa MS, Wright MJ, Hunt JP, et al: Factors affecting the diagnosis and prediction of PTSD symptomatology in children and adolescents. Am J Psychiatry 163:644–651, 2006

Schroeder JM, Polusny MA: Risk factors for adolescent alcohol use following a natural disaster. Prehosp Disaster Med 19:122–127, 2004

Schuster MA, Stein BD, Jaycox L, et al: A national survey of stress reactions after the September 11, 2001, terrorist attacks. N Engl J Med 345:1507–1512, 2001

Shaw JA: Children, adolescents and trauma. Psychiatr Q 71:227–243, 2000

Shaw JA, Applegate B, Tanner S, et al: Psychological effects of Hurricane Andrew on an elementary school population. J Amer Acad Child Adolesc Psychiatry 34:1185–1192, 1995

Shaw JA, Applegate B, Schorr C: Twenty-one-month follow-up study of school-age children exposed to Hurricane Andrew. J Amer Acad Child Adolesc Psychiatry 35:359–364, 1996

Spear L: The developing brain and adolescent-typical behavior patterns: an evolutionary approach, in Adolescent Psychopathology and the Developing Brain. Edited by Romer D, Walker EF. Oxford, UK, Oxford University Press, 2007, pp 9–30

Stover CS, Berkowitz S, Marans S, et al: Posttraumatic stress disorder, in Lewis's Child and Adolescent Psychiatry, in Lewis's Child and Adolescent Psychiatry. Edited by Martin A, Volkmar FR. Philadelphia, PA, Wolters Kluwer, 2007, pp 701–711

Stuber J, Fairbrother G, Galea S, et al: Determinants of counseling for children in Manhattan after the September 11 attacks. Psychiatr Serv 53:815–822, 2002

Terr LC: Forbidden games, posttraumatic child's play. J Am Acad Child Adolesc Psychiatry 20:741–760, 1981a

Terr L: Psychic trauma in children: observations following the Chowchilla school bus kidnappings. Am J Psychiatry 138:14–19, 1981b

Terr L: What happens to early memories of trauma? A study of twenty children under age five at the time of documented traumatic events. J Am Acad Child Adolesc Psychiatry 27:96–104, 1988

Terr L: Childhood traumas: an outline and overview. Am J Psychiatry 148:10–20, 1991

Triffleman EG, Marmar CR, Delucchi KL, et al: Childhood trauma and posttraumatic stress disorder in substance abuse inpatients. J Nerv Ment Dis 183:172–176, 1995

Werner EE, Smith RS: Vulnerable but Invincible: A Study of Resilient Children. New York, McGraw-Hill, 1982

5

Children With Special Needs During Disasters

Introduction

Collectively, children are regarded as a special population, and subgroups of children have additional special needs. Flynn (2006) defined special populations as "groups of people whose needs may require additional, customized, or specialized approaches in preparedness for, response to, and recovery from extreme events" (p. 12), but indicated that "needing attention" does not necessarily signify higher risk. Flynn admonished against equating special population status with higher risk for psychosocial consequences, noting instead that increased risk is associated with some, but not all, special population subgroups. For example, subgroups of persons who do not speak the dominant language of the area require special approaches to disaster preparedness, warning, and response, but these groups may not be at increased risk for medical or psychological disaster consequences.

The following are important points to remember about children with special needs during disasters:

1. Children are themselves a special population.
2. Prior to disaster, there are subgroups of children who have definable special needs and who are vulnerable to disaster-related psychological distress and impairment.
3. Some children with prior special needs who are exposed to disaster may experience exacerbation of their special needs.
4. Some children with no prior special needs may emerge from disaster with special needs.
5. Children who are living in poverty or foster care or who are of minority status may experience more psychosocial consequences in disasters.

Some children will qualify as having "special needs" on the basis of their individual or family health risk history, and this status will be known predisaster. Many of these children will already be receiving targeted treatments and therapies, or possibly special forms of education and community programming. These children may be enrolled in various registries to receive special resources, including, in some instances, individualized planning for disaster evacuation or supportive care.

A critical caveat, however, is that special population "eligibility" is not exclusively predetermined or predefined by predisaster characteristics. Disasters change the world and "reshuffle the deck." When disaster strikes, exposure to the disaster event or to postimpact adversities will transform some child disaster survivors and some entire families that have no predisaster history into persons with special needs. Children who experience various forms of disaster-related injury, psychological trauma, loss, or hardship will emerge with special needs in the aftermath.

Disability refers to personal and medical histories that may include prior trauma, substance abuse, preexisting mental illness, and diminished health status. Populations generally considered to be at "high risk" or vulnerable at the time of disaster include children, the elderly, individuals with limited language proficiency; individuals who are economically disadvantaged or culturally or geographically isolated, and individuals with disabilities. Other demographic characteristics that signify disparities in disaster risk are gender, race, and ethnicity.

Children as a Special Needs Population

This book focuses on children exposed to the traumatizing effects of disasters precisely because children are a special population. Cognizant of the distinctive needs of children, the National Commission on Children and Disasters (NCCD) was empaneled by the U.S. government as an independent federal advisory committee that was instructed "to conduct a comprehensive study to independently examine and assess the needs of children (0–18 years of age) in relation to the preparation for, response to, and recovery from all hazards, including major disasters and emergencies" (NCCD 2010).

In 2010, the NCCD issued its final report, specifying its findings and recommendations in the areas of 1) disaster management and recovery; 2) mental health; 3) child physical health and trauma; 4) emergency medical services and transport; 5) disaster case management; 6) child care and early education; 7) elementary and secondary education; 8) child welfare and juvenile justice; 9) sheltering standards, services, and supplies; 10) housing; and 11) evacuation. The commissioners concluded, "Each new disaster presents distinct challenges. However, we can anticipate the needs of children and, therefore, we can and must prepare to meet those needs." The commission's wide-ranging recommendations (Table 5–1) are a testament to the multifaceted nature of the process required to comprehensively address the special needs of children in disasters.

The NCCD (2010) focused specifically on the mental health needs of children exposed to disasters, echoing the assertions of Schonfeld (2004) that children are not equipped, by virtue of limited experience, skills, and resources, to meet their own mental and behavioral health needs. In addition to children's documented vulnerability for developing disaster-related posttraumatic stress disorder (PTSD), depression, and anxiety disorders, and the likelihood that some children will experience traumatic bereavement due to the loss of loved ones and caregivers in the disaster, children may also experience postdisaster academic failure and behavioral problems such as delinquency and substance abuse (Masten and Osofsky 2010; Pane et al. 2008; Silverman and LaGreca 2002). For example, in a study of children in coastal Louisiana and Mississippi, Abramson et al. (2010), from the National Center for Disaster Preparedness, estimated that the incidence of emotional and behavioral distress that was directly attributable to the Gulf of Mexico oil spill disaster was 19%.

TABLE 5–1. **Recommendations of the National Commission on Children and Disasters**

---

1. Disaster management and recovery

   1.1: Distinguish and comprehensively integrate the needs of children across all inter- and intra-governmental disaster management activities and operations.

   1.2: The President should accelerate the development and implementation of the National Disaster Recovery Framework with an explicit emphasis on addressing the immediate and long-term physical and mental health, educational, housing, and human services recovery needs of children.

   1.3: DHS/FEMA should ensure that information required for timely and effective delivery of recovery services to children and families is collected and shared with appropriate entities.

   1.4: DHS/FEMA should establish interagency agreements to provide disaster preparedness funding, technical assistance, training, and other resources to State and local child serving systems and child congregate care facilities.

2. Mental health

   2.1: HHS should lead efforts to integrate mental and behavioral health for children into public health, medical, and other relevant disaster management activities.

   2.2: HHS should enhance the research agenda for children's disaster mental and behavioral health, including psychological first aid, cognitive-behavioral interventions, social support interventions, bereavement counseling and support, and programs intended to enhance children's resilience in the aftermath of a disaster.

   2.3: Federal agencies and non-Federal partners should enhance pre-disaster preparedness and just-in-time training in pediatric disaster mental and behavioral health, including psychological first aid, bereavement support, and brief supportive interventions, for mental health professionals and individuals, such as teachers, who work with children.

   2.4: DHS/FEMA and SAMHSA should strengthen the Crisis Counseling Assistance and Training Program (CCP) to better meet the mental health needs of children and families.

   2.5: Congress should establish a single, flexible grant funding mechanism to specifically support the delivery of mental health treatment services that address the full spectrum of behavioral health needs of children including treatment of disaster-related adjustment difficulties, psychiatric disorders, and substance abuse.

TABLE 5–1.	Recommendations of the National Commission on Children and Disasters *(continued)*

3. Child physical health and trauma

   3.1: Congress, HHS, and DHS/FEMA should ensure availability of and access to pediatric medical countermeasures (MCM) at the Federal, State, and local levels for chemical, biological, radiological, nuclear, and explosive threats.

   3.2: HHS and DoD should enhance the pediatric capabilities of their disaster medical response teams through the integration of pediatric-specific training, guidance, exercises, supplies, and personnel.

   3.3: HHS should ensure that health professionals who may treat children during a disaster have adequate pediatric disaster clinical training.

   3.4: The Executive Branch and Congress should provide resources for a formal regionalized pediatric system of care to support pediatric surge capacity during and after disasters.

   3.5: Prioritize the recovery of pediatric health and mental health care delivery systems in disaster-affected areas.

   3.6: EPA should engage State and local health officials and non-governmental experts to develop and promote national guidance and best practices on re-occupancy of homes, schools, child care, and other child congregate care facilities in disaster-impacted areas.

4. Emergency medical services and pediatric transport

   4.1: The President and Congress should clearly designate and appropriately resource a lead Federal agency for emergency medical services (EMS) with primary responsibility for the coordination of grant programs, research, policy, and standards development and implementation.

   4.2: Improve the capability of emergency medical services (EMS) to transport pediatric patients and provide comprehensive pre-hospital pediatric care during daily operations and disasters.

   4.3: HHS should develop a national strategy to improve Federal pediatric emergency transport and patient care capabilities for disasters.

TABLE 5–1.	Recommendations of the National Commission on Children and Disasters *(continued)*

5. Disaster case management

    5.1: Disaster case management programs should be appropriately resourced and should provide consistent holistic services that achieve tangible, positive outcomes for children and families affected by the disaster.

6. Child care and early education

    6.1: Congress and HHS should improve disaster preparedness capabilities for childcare.

    6.2: Congress and Federal agencies should improve capacity to provide childcare services in the immediate aftermath of and recovery from a disaster.

    6.3: HHS should require disaster preparedness capabilities for Head Start Centers and basic disaster mental health training for staff.

7. Elementary and secondary education

    7.1: Congress and Federal agencies should improve the preparedness of schools and school districts by providing additional support to States.

    7.2: Congress and ED should enhance the ability of school personnel to support children who are traumatized, grieving, or otherwise recovering from a disaster.

    7.3: Ensure that school systems recovering from disasters are provided immediate resources to reopen and restore the learning environment in a timely manner and provide support for displaced students and their host schools.

8. Child welfare and juvenile justice

    8.1: Ensure that State and local child welfare agencies adequately prepare for disasters.

    8.2: Ensure that State and local juvenile justice agencies and all residential treatment, correctional, and detention facilities that house children adequately prepare for disasters.

    8.3: HHS and DOJ should ensure that juvenile, dependency, and other courts hearing matters involving children adequately prepare for disasters.

TABLE 5–1. Recommendations of the National Commission on Children and Disasters (*continued*)

9. Sheltering standards, services, and supplies

 9.1: Government agencies and non-governmental organizations should provide a safe and secure mass care shelter environment for children, including access to essential services and supplies.

10. Housing

 10.1: Prioritize the needs of families with children, especially families with children who have disabilities or chronic health, mental health, or educational needs, within disaster housing assistance programs.

11. Evacuation

 11.1: Congress and Federal agencies should provide sufficient funding to develop and deploy a national information sharing capability to quickly and effectively reunite displaced children with their families, guardians, and caregivers when separated by a disaster.

 11.2: Disaster plans at all levels of government must specifically address the evacuation and transportation needs of children with disabilities and chronic health needs, in coordination with child congregate care facilities such as schools, childcare, and health care facilities.

Note. DHS=Department of Homeland Security; DoD=Department of Defense; DOJ=Department of Justice; ED=Department of Education; EPA=Environmental Protection Agency; FEMA=Federal Emergency Management Agency; HHS=Department of Health and Human Services; SAMHSA=Substance Abuse and Mental Health Services Administration.
Source. Reprinted from National Commission on Children and Disasters: *2010 Report to the President and Congress* (AHRQ Publication No. 10-M037). Rockville, MD, Agency for Healthcare Research and Quality, 2010.

Children With Acute and Chronic Medical Problems

Children with chronic medical needs, severe acute illness, or serious injury may encounter extraordinary barriers to care and challenges to survival in disaster situations, especially when disaster strikes with minimal warning (Cohen 2000). Some children require life-sustaining care during disasters; these include newborns, children in intensive care, children with critical medical conditions, those who require life-supporting medications (e.g., insulin for diabetes, inhalers for asthma) or medical treatments (e.g., kidney dialysis), those who are dependent on oxygen or electric life-support equipment, those with immunosuppression, and those whose illnesses or injuries keep them immobilized. Children with chronic medical conditions can be identified and registered to receive special transport and care during times of disaster. At any moment, however, other children may be hospitalized for acute, life-threatening illness, and they will also be at elevated risk should disaster strike. In the case of a pandemic disease, such as severe influenza, large numbers of children may be at extreme risk simultaneously. The American Psychiatric Association (2007) has provided a detailed spectrum of children with special needs (Table 5–2).

Children With Disabilities

Children compromised by disabilities include those with visual and hearing impairments, mobility impairments, chronic illnesses, developmental disabilities, brain injuries, drug and/or alcohol dependence, mental illness, and dual diagnoses of mental illness and substance abuse. The disability category also subsumes those children who use life-support systems, depend on service animals, and are medically dependent on others for sustained care.

Individuals with disabilities make up a sizable portion of the general population of the United States. The National Council on Disability (2005) indicated that disabled persons constitute 19.3% of U.S. citizens, age 5 years and older, in the civilian noninstitutionalized population. Children who have sensory disabilities (i.e., those who are blind, deaf, and hard of hearing) or motor disabilities, as well as those who have high-risk or chronic health conditions that affect mobility or make them dependent on electric equipment or electronic devices, are the most recognizable subgroups. Less recognized are children with cognitive disabilities, who may present particular challenges in large-scale emergencies due to their potential difficulty with understanding and following directions, which could place them and others in harm's way. Children with learning and language disabilities or limitations of intellectual skills are likewise at increased risk for harm.

"Vulnerable" or "at risk" children and their families may not be able to avail themselves of the usual resources for disaster preparedness, relief, recovery, and mitigation. Families with children who have disabilities

TABLE 5–2.   Children with special needs

Children with developmental disabilities	**Children who experience cultural/ethnic health disparities or live in geographic isolation**
Blind and visually impaired	Cultural/ethnic groups
Deaf and hard of hearing	Rural residents
Mobility impaired	**Children with limited language proficiency**
Mentally ill	Limited-English or non-English speaking
Brain disorders and injuries	Refugees
Chronically ill	Legal immigrants
Drug and/or alcohol dependent	Illegal/undocumented immigrants
Dually diagnosed with mental illness and substance abuse	Sign language
Children with special psychiatric needs	**Children exposed to maltreatment**
Children who were previously defined as psychiatrically disturbed, and/or who were receiving psychotropic medication, and/or whose condition worsened due to the lack of access to medications	Physical abuse
	Emotional abuse
Children with preexisting psychosocial and psychiatric problems which are exacerbated by the stress of disaster	Neglect
	Sexual abuse
Children with special medical needs	**Others**
Children with medical needs	Juvenile offenders
Families with children with medical needs	Dependent on public transportation
Children who live in economic disadvantage	Families underserved by public health
Population-wide poverty	Sheltered juveniles: runaways, battered youth
Living at or below the poverty line	Homeless youth
Working poor	

Source.   Adapted from American Psychiatric Association 2007.

and activity limitations will need to preplan and activate their disaster preparedness and mitigation activities (e.g., installing hurricane shutters, sheltering, evacuating) much earlier than their counterparts who have no family members with special needs.

Developmental disability is defined as physical or mental disability, or a combination of both, that is continuous and manifest during childhood. Developmental disability is frequently evidenced by limitations in expressive and receptive language, self-care, learning, mobility, and capacity for independent living. The population prevalence of developmental disability is 2%–3%. Developmental disabilities may derive from a diversity of origins: congenital malformations; birth injuries; brain injuries; and chronic medical illnesses such as cystic fibrosis, HIV infection, diabetes, and neurological disabilities. Children with developmental disabilities are more likely to be abused. Abuse, in turn, precipitates further developmental delays across social, psychological, physical, and cognitive domains. Ongoing and repetitive episodes of trauma sustained by children with developmental disabilities increase the children's vulnerability when they confront a natural or human-generated disaster.

Compared with nondisabled members of the population, people with disabilities have notably increased apprehension about the future occurrence of disasters and emergencies (White et al. 2004). Their concerns are well founded because disaster preparedness and emergency response systems are typically designed for people without disabilities, for whom escape or rescue involves walking, running, driving, seeing, hearing, and quickly responding to directions (White et al. 2004).

Children With Psychiatric Needs

Adverse psychological reactions during disasters are more common for persons who have been diagnosed with severe and persistent mental illness, previous history of trauma, psychiatric diagnosis, and history of substance abuse (Norris et al. 2002). Much of the documentation for this finding comes from studies of adults. For example, in the aftermath of the Madrid railway bombing in 2004, both disaster-associated PTSD and major depression were found to be strongly associated with a history of diagnosable psychiatric disorder (Gabriel et al. 2007). Survivors of the 1995 Oklahoma City bombing who had a history of psychiatric disorder had twice the rate of event-associated PTSD compared with survivors with no prior disorder (North et al. 1999). Corroborating findings were found for survivors of the September 11, 2001, attacks on

America (Boscarino et al. 2003) and the 1991 Oakland/Berkeley, California, firestorm (Koopman et al. 1994); in both cases, prior psychiatric history strongly predicted disaster-associated PTSD. Researchers have noted that persons with a prior psychiatric diagnosis (PTSD, depression, anxiety disorder, substance abuse disorder) are more vulnerable to new trauma because of their diminished abilities to cope with the escalating demands that occur in situations of disaster or terrorism (Franklin et al. 2002; Hobfoll et al. 2006).

Families with members who have special psychiatric needs face systemic challenges. Following Hurricane Katrina, the National Organization on Disability (2005) released a critical report focusing on the emergency response for an estimated 65,000 persons in New Orleans with a mental disability. Their conclusion was powerful: "People with psychiatric disabilities were discriminated against during evacuation, rescue, and relief phases" (p. 3). Many residents were not evacuated and were prevented from entering shelter facilities or were physically segregated. Others who were evacuated were dispersed to distant states without a tracking system or support resources. Clients were separated from mental health professionals and community mental health centers with no mechanism for tracking them. Psychiatric treatment sites and medications were unavailable for many residents, and other residents were inappropriately admitted to nursing home facilities and institutionalized care.

Children in Foster Care

The U.S. welfare system subsumes a complex matrix of services and programs, which vary by state and across communities (Grigsby 2002). Children who are placed in foster care have usually experienced neglect and physical, emotional, and/or sexual abuse. These children have frequently experienced a myriad of stressors within the family, including mental disorders, substance abuse, domestic violence, financial hardships, chronic medical illness, and death of loved ones. Environmental stressors may include racial and ethnic discrimination, unemployment, and poverty.

The foster care population in the United States is estimated to number about 500,000; children reside in a variety of settings, such as youth shelters, group homes, domestic violence shelters, residential treatment centers, and foster homes. Children in foster care have higher rates of child maltreatment and psychiatric disorders. The high prevalence of previous trauma increases the vulnerability and diminishes the resilience of foster children when they are subsequently exposed to disasters and extreme events.

Hurricane Katrina brought the vulnerabilities of foster care children into sharp focus. Many of the 13,000 children who were in foster care in Louisiana, Alabama, and Mississippi prior to storm impact were displaced after the storm. These children frequently experienced separations from adult caretakers and the other foster care children with whom they were living at the time of storm impact. Displacement and relocation of foster children disrupted their schooling and friendship networks. Those who were resettled to other states often lost their eligibility to receive the welfare and Medicaid benefits from their state of origin (Gelles 2006).

Children of Minorities

In Chapter 3, "The Context of Trauma," we discussed issues of race, ethnicity, and minority status, with particular emphasis on observed disparities in risk and access to disaster services. Here, we revisit this important topic in the context of special needs. As Hawkins et al. (2009) stated,

> Marginalized populations, most notably racial/ethnic minorities and individuals with low socioeconomic status (SES), are at heightened risk for disaster exposure and vulnerability to disaster-related mental health outcomes.... Marginalized populations are most often defined by race/ethnicity, SES, geography, gender, age, and disability status. In disaster research, marginalized populations refer to individuals within these categories who are disproportionately affected by disaster and are most vulnerable to negative consequences of disaster. (p. 277)

Minority status may confer increased risk in disasters but also may introduce important protective factors. Well publicized is the finding of significantly higher rates of posttraumatic stress symptoms among New York City Hispanic residents, compared with non-Hispanics, who responded to a population survey conducted after the September 11 attack (Galea et al. 2004). Following Hurricane Katrina, racial and ethnic minority disaster survivors perceived that they had been left in harm's way without means to protect their neighborhoods or to evacuate to safety and that both emergency response and recovery operations were delayed because of the survivors' minority status (Bourque et al. 2006; Eisenman et al. 2007; Weems et al. 2007). The literature on social support among minority populations in relation to disaster risk is mixed.

Some studies have documented heightened risk for some groups (Hawkins et al. 2009), whereas other studies have found that the family, social, and spiritual support within some minority populations may exert a beneficial effect on individuals' mental health in the aftermath of disaster (Bauer et al. 2000; Constantine et al. 2005). Implications for children are evident: to the extent that disaster risk, disaster-related behaviors (preparedness, evacuation, sheltering), availability of emergency services, access to recovery resources, and community social support differ based on minority status, these differences will have direct bearing on the mental and behavioral health of families and children.

Children With Disaster-Related Special Needs

All disasters disrupt family and community function, but more so for those families and communities with serious preexisting problems. In addition, experiencing the forces of harm during disaster impact is a transforming event. Many disaster survivors, including children and their caregivers, regardless of preimpact status, will emerge distressed and fearful. Most will recover fairly rapidly with appropriate family and social supports. However, depending on the balance of exposure, risk, and protective factors, some children may ultimately require a more sustained psychosocial intervention. Children with fewer personal and family resources to facilitate recovery may need more customized or tailored support and intervention.

In some instances, an encounter with disaster will create new and possibly urgent special needs for children and families who previously had none. For example, some healthy, athletic children will be severely injured and suddenly require emergency care and sophisticated medical or surgical intervention. Some may incur life-changing injuries. Other children will be uninjured but will be severely traumatized. Some children may lose a parent in the disaster; in fact, during catastrophic events and pandemics, children may be orphaned. The combination of both traumatic loss and financial hardship when the family breadwinner is suddenly killed may precipitate urgent and acute special needs.

Because of the havoc of disaster and flawed logistics, some otherwise healthy children end up having special needs. For example, during Hurricane Katrina, more than 5,000 children became separated from their parents during the evacuation process (Broughton et al. 2006; Chung and Shannon 2007).

Interventions
Predisaster Phase

Children with special needs require medical and community interventions that are mobilized to ensure the safety and protection of each child. These interventions include child protective services, medical care venues, foster care placement, and residential care when indicated. Children with identified special needs are usually in an ongoing intervention program prior to the occurrence of a disaster in their community. Because programs for special needs children are multifaceted and time phased, continuity of care is essential for optimal outcomes; this requires a sustained investment of resources and planning for continuity of operations during extreme events. Predisaster planning must prioritize support for the entire family with a special needs child because optimal therapeutic outcome is closely tied to parental and family influences.

In the preimpact phase, efforts should be made by both municipal and mental health professionals to promote community contingency plans for children who have been exposed to cumulative traumatic experiences and who will need to have special consideration at the time of disaster. Parents need to prepare for the eventuality of emergency situations such as disasters that may interfere with the continuity of health care, family stability, and social supports. Families need to be informed about the potential hazards that are likely to occur in the local area. They benefit from anticipating and preparing for such emergencies by becoming informed about community disaster and evacuation plans, school plans for reuniting children and families at the time of disaster, and the locations of special needs shelters. Parents are encouraged to develop alliances with health care providers, to prepare emergency supply kits with the child's critical medical supplies and necessary medications, and to have contingency plans to request and receive assistance from other family members in time of need.

Families are strongly encouraged to create a family disaster plan with the active participation of all family members and ideally to conduct family disaster drills based on those plans. Completing the family disaster plan will require some budgeting and some shopping over a period of weeks or months to accrue a family stockpile of emergency supplies and "go kits" (personal emergency kits) for every member of the family. Particularly critical, especially for families with special needs children, is to have a family communications plan to maintain or, if necessary, reestablish communications among family members when a disaster warning is issued or an unexpected emergency occurs. In particular, families with

TABLE 5–3.	Disaster plan recommendations for caregivers of children with special health needs

Have a clearly defined disaster care plan for child.

Develop strong alliances with health care providers.

Maintain phone numbers of health providers.

Know the location of emergency health centers.

Have a medical supplies kit tailored to the needs of the child.

Obtain medical identification tags for your child.

Train family members to assume the role of in-home health care providers.

Identify a common point of contact (neighbor, friend, or relative) in the event that family members are separated.

Identify an out-of-state contact person in the event that local communications are disrupted.

Stockpile foods that are essential for special dietary needs or restrictions.

Learn the disaster plan at the child's school, including how the school plans to reunite children and families if a disaster strikes during school hours.

Know where evacuation shelters are located.

Learn the community's evacuation routes.

For children with medical conditions requiring electrical power, notify utility companies to provide emergency support during a disaster.

Identify shelters in the area that provide continuous power during disasters.

Create contingency plans should the utility company not be able to provide alternative sources of power in the event of power loss.

Evacuate when told to do so.

Source. Adapted from Markenson and Reynolds 2006.

special needs children must plan for earlier and timely evacuation (Peek and Stough 2010). Recommendations for caregivers of children with special needs are provided in Table 5–3.

Impact Phase

During disaster impact, children in harm's way are exposed to a range of stressors. This is the time to put into operation the family's emergency plans for ensuring safety from the disaster, continuing health care, and family stability. Because previous exposure to psychosocial adversities increases the vulnerability for additional traumatic exposure, special needs children should be prioritized for evacuation to safe environments with ongoing provision of services, with the goal of minimizing the intensity of exposure and the disruption of care.

When a disaster occurs, children may be harmed and traumatized, loved ones may be injured or killed, and the impacts on family and community will disrupt lifestyle routines. The NCCD's (2010) recommendations, listed in Table 5–1, will be effective in diminishing the medical, psychological, and social consequences for children exposed to disaster. These suggestions include prioritization of the children's needs when devising community disaster management plans coupled with rapid implementation of the National Disaster Recovery Framework in a manner that addresses children's immediate and long-term needs related to physical and mental health, education, housing, and human services.

Specific to the mental health and psychosocial support needs of children impacted by disaster, the NCCD recommendations include 1) integration of mental and behavioral health with medical and public health interventions for disaster-affected families; 2) use of a stepped-care approach to provide community-level psychosocial support, brief supportive interventions at the family level, and individualized psychological or psychiatric intervention as needed with disaster-impacted children; 3) activation of the Crisis Counseling Assistance and Training Program to bring mental health resources to disaster-affected communities; and 4) long-term provision of "mental health treatment services that address the full spectrum of behavioral health needs of children including treatment of disaster-related adjustment difficulties, psychiatric disorders, and substance abuse" (NCCD 2010).

Postdisaster Phase

Several factors in the postdisaster recovery period may exacerbate psychosocial stressors on children and their families and impede recovery. These include complicated bereavement, loss of social supports, loss of resources, and damage to community and family function (Shultz et al. 2007a).

Social support is an extremely important buffer against the traumatizing effects of disaster (Kaniasty 2005). Conversely, lack of social support is one of the most robust predictors of disaster-related PTSD (Brewin 2001). Loss of community and social support systems is viewed as one of the most powerful predictors of psychological morbidities secondary to disaster exposures (Hobfoll et al. 2006). Subsequent to disaster, community infrastructure may be in disarray, compromising virtually all systems of care ordinarily available to citizens. Children with special needs will be most profoundly affected by the interruption or loss of critical services.

Following a disaster's impact, the focus for special needs children should be on maintaining or rapidly restoring supportive services and care environments. Accurate assessment of the child's symptoms facilitates tailored and customized intervention as needed in the aftermath of the disaster experience. Every effort should be made to enhance the child's coping capacities and resilience, and to mitigate the child's uncertainty, physical discomfort, and perception of social isolation or separation from loved ones.

Particular attention should be given to providing disaster recovery and behavioral health support for the parents and caregivers of special needs children. The parents' management of essential care is critical for mitigating the traumatic events for the children. However, as disaster survivors themselves, the parents also need all manner of available support.

Assessment and intervention at the time of disaster impact and its aftermath must be sensitized to culturally competent practices. A traumatic event is interpreted and given meaning within the context of ethnic and cultural values and beliefs. During disasters, care and support must be provided to disaster-affected populations that reflect a mix of cultures, value systems, health beliefs, and primary languages.

Postdisaster helpers need to assess each child's and family's level of acculturation and corresponding level of "acculturative stress." For example, a child may feel comfortable speaking English and be more acculturated than the parents, who may prefer to speak their native language. When possible, an interpreter or a provider who is fluent in the family's native language should be involved. A culturally competent needs assessment will address issues of cultural identity, values and health beliefs, treatment expectations, family supports, cross-generational differences in acculturation, and trauma associated with migration and relocation. It is important to perceive the child as part of the family unit and to engage the family as a whole. For example, the centrality of family within the Hispanic community requires that helpers recognize the importance of engaging the entire family in any assessment or integration process.

■ Key Clinical Points

- ■ Children are themselves a special population.

- ■ Prior to disaster, there are subgroups of children who have definable special needs and who are vulnerable to disaster-related psychological distress and impairment.

- ■ Some children with prior special needs who are exposed to disaster may experience exacerbation of their special needs.

- ■ Some children with no prior special needs may emerge from disaster with special needs due to the effects of the disaster.

- ■ Children living in poverty or children of minority status may experience more psychosocial consequences in disasters.

- ■ Interventions for children with special needs require preimpact planning.

- ■ Interventions during the impact phase and postrecovery phase require mobilization of community and health care response systems that are attentive to children with special needs.

References

Abramson D, Redlener I, Stehling-Ariza T, et al: Impact on Children and Families of the Deepwater Horizon Oil Spill: Preliminary Findings of the Coastal Population Impact Study (Research Brief 2010:8). August 3, 2010. New York, National Center for Disaster Preparedness, Columbia University, Mailman School of Public Health. Available at: www.ncdp.mailman. columbia.edu/files/NCDP_Oil_Impact_Report.pdf. Accessed August 29, 2011.

American Psychiatric Association: Special Populations. 2007. Available at: www.psych.org/disaster/dpc_populations.cfm.

Bauer H, Rodriguez M, Quiroga S, et al: Barriers to health care for abused Latina and Asian immigrant women. J Health Care Poor Underserved 11:33–44, 2000

Boscarino JA, Galea S, Ahern J, et al: Psychiatric medication use among Manhattan residents following the World Trade Center disaster. J Trauma Stress 16:301–306, 2003

Bourque L, Siegel J, Kano M, et al: Weathering the storm: the impact of hurricanes on physical and mental health. Ann Am Acad Pol Soc Sci 604:129–151, 2006

Brewin C: Cognitive and emotional reactions to traumatic events: implications for short-term intervention. Adv Mind Body Med 17:163–168, 2001

Broughton DD, Allen EE, Hannemann RE, et al: Getting 5000 families back together: reuniting fractured families after a disaster: the role of the National Center for Missing and Exploited Children. Pediatrics 117:S442–S445, 2006

Chung S, Shannon M: Reuniting children with their families during disasters: a proposed plan for greater success. Am J Disaster Med 2:113–117, 2007

Cohen R: Mental Health Services in Disasters: Manual for Humanitarian Workers. Washington, DC, Pan-American Health Organization, 2000

Constantine MG, Alleyne VL, Caldwell LD, et al: Coping responses of Asian, black, and Latino/Latina New York City residents following the September 11, 2001 terrorist attacks against the United States. Cultur Divers Ethnic Minor Psychol 11:293–308, 2005

Eisenman D, Cordasco K, Asch S, et al: Disaster planning and risk communication with vulnerable communities: lessons learned from Hurricane Katrina. Am J Public Health 97:S109–S115, 2007

Flynn BW: Meeting the needs of special populations in disasters and emergencies: making it work in rural areas. Paper presented at the annual meeting of the National Association for Rural Mental Health, San Antonio, TX, August 2006

Franklin CL, Young D, Zimmerman M: Psychiatric patients' vulnerability in the wake of the September 11th terrorist attacks. J Nerv Ment Dis 190:833–838, 2002

Gabriel R, Ferrando L, Cortón ES, et al: Psychopathological consequences after a terrorist attack: an epidemiological study among victims, the general population, and police officers. Eur Psychiatry 22:339–346, 2007

Galea S, Vlahov D, Tracy M, et al: Hispanic ethnicity and post-traumatic stress disorder after a disaster: evidence from a general population survey after September 11, 2001. Ann Epidemiol 14:520–531, 2004

Gelles RJ: Responding to the Needs of the Lost and Forgotten: Foster Children and Battered Women Before and After Hurricane Katrina. 2006. Available at: www.sp2.upenn.edu/fieldctr/newsletters/spring2006/responding.html. Accessed August 31, 2011.

Grigsby RK: Consultation with foster care homes, group homes, youth shelters, domestic violence shelters, and big brothers and big sister programs, in Child and Adolescent Psychiatry. Edited by Lewis M. New York, Lippincott Williams & Wilkins, 2002

Hawkins AO, Zinzow HM, Amstadter AB, et al: Factors associated with response to disasters among marginalized populations, in Mental Health and Disasters. Edited by Neria Y, Galea S, Norris FH. Cambridge, UK, Cambridge University Press, 2009, pp 277–290

Hobfoll SE, Tracy M, Galea S: The impact of resource loss and traumatic growth on probable PTSD and depression following terrorist attacks. J Trauma Stress 19:867–878, 2006

Kaniasty K: Social support and traumatic stress. National Center for Post-Traumatic Stress Disorder PTSD Research Quarterly 16:1–7, 2005

Koopman C, Classen C, Spiegel D: Predictors of posttraumatic stress symptoms among survivors of the Oakland/Berkeley, California, firestorm. Am J Psychiatry 151:888–894, 1994

Markenson D, Reynolds S; American Academy of Pediatrics Committee on Pediatric Emergency Medicine; Task Force on Terrorism. The pediatrician and disaster preparedness. Pediatrics 117:e340–e362, 2006

Masten AS, Osofsky JD: Disasters and their impact on child development: introduction to the special section. Child Dev 81:1029–1039, 2010

National Commission on Children and Disasters: 2010 Report to the President and Congress (AHRQ Publ No 10-M037). Rockville, MD, Agency for Healthcare Research and Quality, 2010. Available at: http://archive.ahrq.gov/prep/nccdreport/nccdreport.pdf. Accessed August 29, 2011.

National Council on Disability: Saving Lives: Including People with Disabilities in Emergency Planning. April 15, 2005. Available at: www.ncd.gov/publications/2005/04152005-1. Accessed August 29, 2011.

National Organization on Disability: Polling Data Show People With Disabilities Unprepared for Terrorist, Other Crises at Home or at Work. 2002. Available at: www.nod.org/index.cfm?id=773.

National Organization on Disability: Report on Special Needs Assessment for Katrina Evacuees (SNAKE) Project. Washington, DC, National Organization on Disability, 2006. Available at: http://www.nod.org/assets/downloads/Special-Needs-For-Katrina-Evacuees.doc. Accessed November 9, 2011.

Norris F, Friedman M, Watson P, et al: 60,000 disaster victims speak, part 1: an empirical review of the empirical literature, 1981–2001. Psychiatry 65:207–239, 2002

North CS, Nixon SJ, Shariat S, et al: Psychiatric disorders among survivors of the Oklahoma City bombing. JAMA 282:755–762, 1999

Pane JF, McCaffrey DF, Kalra N, et al: Effects of student displacement in Louisiana during the first academic year after the hurricanes of 2005. Journal of Education for Students Placed at Risk 13:168–211, 2008. Available at: www.rand.org/pubs/reprints/2008/RAND_RP1379.pdf. Accessed August 29, 2011.

Peek L, Stough LM: Children with disabilities in the context of disaster: a social vulnerability perspective. Child Dev 81:1260–1270, 2010

Shultz JM, Espinel Z, Flynn BW, et al: All-Hazards Disaster Behavioral Health Training. Tampa, FL, Disaster Life Support Publishing, 2007a

Shultz JM, Espinel Z, Galea S, et al: Disaster ecology: implications for disaster psychiatry, in Textbook of Disaster Psychiatry. Edited by Ursano RJ, Fullerton CS, Weisaeth L, et al. Cambridge, UK, Cambridge University Press, 2007b, pp 69–96

Silverman WK, LaGreca AM: Children experiencing disasters: definitions, reactions, and predictions of outcomes, in Helping Children Cope With Disasters and Terrorism. Edited by LaGreca AM, Silverman WK, Vernberg EM, et al. Washington, DC, American Psychological Association, 2002, pp 11–33

Weems CF, Watts SE, Marsee MA, et al: The psychosocial impact of Hurricane Katrina: contextual differences in psychological symptoms, social support, and discrimination. Behav Res Ther 45:2295–2306, 2007

White G, Fox M, Rowland J, et al: Nobody Left Behind: Investigating Disaster Preparedness and Response for People With Disabilities. PowerPoint presentation at the National Advisory Board Meeting, Lawrence, KS, May 24, 2004

6

Traumatic Bereavement

Introduction

Children exposed to disaster may experience the death of a parent or other family members or loved ones. Death from disaster usually occurs suddenly and unexpectedly, striking down the healthy and taking life prematurely. *Bereavement* can be defined as the fact of loss through death. Bereavement reactions include both psychological and physiological responses to bereavement. *Grief* refers to the emotions associated with bereavement. *Mourning* is the social expression of grief. Bereavement is usually associated with some symptoms comparable to depression, such as sadness, insomnia, poor appetite, and weight loss, but the bereaved usually experience their responses as normal. The expected duration and expression of grief is determined somewhat by cultural expectations.

Children and Bereavement

Four percent of children younger than age 15 in the United States have experienced the death of a parent (National Center for Health Statistics 1997). The early death of a parent most frequently occurs as the result of trauma. Children are twice as likely to lose their father as to lose their mother. Although less traumatic, the loss of other family members (e.g., siblings or grandparents) or loved ones also may have an enduring psychological effect on the developing child.

Children's early exposure to death—along with the discovery that life is not permanent, the realization that the body is susceptible to harm, and the recognition that one can lose the protective caregiving relationships in their daily lives—is traumatic. Children may suffer not only from the premature loss of a family member, but also from exposure to the cruel and violent nature of the death. Because of their cognitive, emotional, and physical immaturity, children process psychological and physiological reactions to bereavement differently than adults do.

The death of a significant person is among the most stressful events that a young person can experience. A child who has lost a parent, sibling, or other loved one must find a way to cope with the immediate impact of the death on his or her life. Simultaneously, the child must begin the process of mourning and resume normal everyday activities. Adults in the child's life, often in the midst of their own grief, are frequently confused and uncertain about how to respond supportively to a child. The task of the surviving parent or other caretakers is to facilitate the child's process of coping, mourning, and resuming normal life activities.

Children's bereavement responses are shaped by such factors as age, gender, psychological and emotional maturity, adaptive and coping strategies, social supports, circumstances of death, previous experiences with death, relationship to the deceased, and available social support systems (Dowdney 2000). Children who experience the death of a parent usually have several concerns: they do not understand chance happenings and tend to look for sources of blame; they begin to fear that if death happened to someone close to them, death might happen to them; and they experience an increasing sense of vulnerability and concerns about abandonment, which make them wonder who is going to take care of them and provide support.

Although children do not usually experience intense or prolonged emotional and behavioral grief reactions, their mourning processes usually last longer than those of adults. For example, parent bereavement over the loss of a child is a process that continues over time, whereas children who experience parental loss often experience thoughts and emotions related to the loss during life's milestones and transitions, such as when they go away to camp or school, receive recognition for achievements, graduate, get married, or give birth to their own children.

Disaster and Child Traumatic Grief

Most studies have concentrated on the responses of adults to disaster-related loss. More than 3,000 people lost their lives in the September 11, 2001, attacks on America. Approximately 11%–14% of adults in New York City lost a friend or relative (Neria et al. 2007). Prigerson et al. (1997) demonstrated that bereavement associated with traumatic grief increases the risk for subsequent mental and physical morbidity. One year after the September 11 attacks, a systematic survey of 929 adults in New York City found that 25% knew someone who was killed, and these individuals were two times more likely than a comparison group to screen positive for a mental disorder such as depression, generalized anxiety disorder, and posttraumatic stress disorder (PTSD) (Neria et al. 2007).

Pynoos et al. (1987) evaluated school-age children 1 year after a school shooting and found that grief symptoms were more persistent than symptoms of PTSD. Adolescents who lost a family member in the 2004 Indian Ocean tsunami were found to have significantly increased risk for depression and PTSD (Wickrama and Kaspar 2007). Pfefferbaum et al. (2006) studied children who had lost a parent, relative, or friend in the 1998 U.S. Embassy bombing in Nairobi, Kenya, and found that 8–14 months after the event, those who had lost a parent had more severe posttraumatic stress symptoms.

There is increasing awareness that child traumatic grief is different from normal bereavement. In childhood traumatic grief, the bereavement process is interwoven with the experience of trauma such that the normal mourning process becomes confounded with issues of posttraumatic stress symptoms and the attempt to resolve traumatic grief. The interaction of grief symptoms with the trauma experience means that memories of the loved one may become confounded with traumatic images of how the individual died. This reliving can be precipitated by traumatic reminders that bring back to conscious awareness all the elements of the traumatic experience. Memories may resurface secondary to life experiences that should have been shared with the departed, such as graduation or other social events. Some common responses associated with child traumatic grief are noted in Table 6–1.

TABLE 6–1.	Common responses in child traumatic grief	
Thoughts	Paradoxical intrusive thoughts and images of traumatic death and avoidance of thoughts/images	Decreased concentration Dissociative responses
	Images of horror	
Emotions	Longing for security/safety	Yearning for lost person
	Intense anxiety	Helplessness
	Fears of recurrence	Separation anxiety
	Anger, irritability, and sadness	
	Frozen emotionality	
Physiological reactions	Acute stress response	Searching behavior
	Hyperarousal	Disorganized behaviors
	Exaggerated startle reactions	Somatic ills

Parent Bereavement

A parent's loss of a child is particularly poignant. Both the Oklahoma City bombing and the September 11 World Trade Center bombing resulted in the tragic deaths of children. When a child dies as a result of trauma, a parent's grief may be confounded with posttraumatic stress reactions (Breslau et al. 1998). The discovery that one's child is prematurely ripped away from the family leaves the parent with a pervasive feeling of despair and emptiness. The grief of parents following the loss of a child is more intense and prolonged than grief following other losses (Raphael 2006). Parents are at increased risk for suicidal behavior in the month following such a loss and for enduring symptoms of depression and anxiety. Parents in the process of bereavement are understandably preoccupied and withdrawn. An adolescent girl noted that after the death of her maternal grandmother her mother quit talking to her, stopped cooking, and was "not there for me."

Death of a Sibling

The death of a sibling can cause immediate and long-lasting emotional and behavioral effects on children. The death represents the loss of a peer relationship complicated by the special and ambivalent bond between siblings. Siblings share a unique relationship in that they have the same parents and have shared confidences separate from those shared with their parents. The surviving child may experience feelings of guilt associated with sibling rivalry or may harbor feelings of blame that the parents failed to protect the sibling from death. When the loss of a sibling leaves the surviving sibling as an only child, the bereavement experience is particularly difficult.

Worden and Silverman (1996) suggested that the loss of a child in a family carries emotional and behavioral effects on the parenting of the remaining children. Parents may become overprotective of the remaining children. They may also burden the surviving children with a "replacement child script" in which expectations envisioned for the now-deceased child are imposed on the remaining siblings.

Developmental Effects

A child's understanding of death is greatly influenced by cognitive development (Spence and Brent 1984). The interrelationship between the child's understanding of death and grief responses, by age, is detailed in Table 6–2. Notably, even children with age-appropriate bereavement reactions may experience a relapse or exacerbation when confronted with subsequent stressors, symbolic reminders, or additional losses. The bereavement process is a long-lasting and continuing struggle to achieve emotional resolution.

Preschool Child

Generally, younger children may confuse death with going to sleep, or they may think of death as a journey and expect the lost loved one to return. The preschool child is unable to understand death and will manifest distress in behaviors and bodily complaints. The child may exhibit clinging and dependent behaviors, loss of previous developmental achievements such as bowel and bladder control, inattention, disorganized behaviors, tantrums, bodily symptoms, sleep and appetite disturbances, and a variety of other anxiety and mood symptoms.

School-Age Child

The school-age child often imagines death as a ghost or a man on a black horse and fears being hurt. Death is seen as frightening and as

TABLE 6–2. Children's understanding of death and expressions of grief

Age	Understanding of death	Expressions of grief
Infancy	Awareness of absence	Quietness, irritability, decreased activity, poor sleep, and eating disturbance
2–4 years	Death is like sleeping Death is reversible, and the dead can come back to life and be reunited with the bereaved	Problems in eating, sleeping, and bladder and bowel control Fear of abandonment Irritability Self-attributions Egocentric thinking that child did something or thought something that caused the loved person to die or go away
5–6 years	Death is perceived as an iconic fearful dark man on a horse, the grim reaper, ghost, or bogeyman Death is equated with killing Death is final and frightening Denial: death happens to others	Curiosity about death Death as aggressive assault Concerns about imaginary illnesses Feelings of abandonment
7–8 years and older	Death is inevitable Death is final and irreversible Child knows he or she is vulnerable to death	Heightened emotions, guilt, anger, and shame Death anxiety Mood symptoms Changes in eating habits Sleep problems Social withdrawal Impulsive behaviors Survivor guilt Behavior problems Self-attributions

something that happens to older persons. By age 7 or 8, children have some understanding of the finality, inevitability, and irreversibility of death. The child may manifest anxiety, abandonment fears, depressed mood, academic and learning problems, social withdrawal, sleep and appetite disturbances, and a range of behavioral problems. Boys are more likely than girls to express their grief through hyperactivity and aggression and appear to be more vulnerable to the psychological effects of early parent death (Dowdney 2000).

Adolescent

The adolescent may experience a sense of social estrangement, fears of early death, anxiety and mood symptoms, somatic ills, anger, guilt, and behavioral problems. Adolescents may take flight into the pursuit of pleasurable experiences or become more socially withdrawn and narrow the scope of life.

Stages of Bereavement

Psychological responses to bereavement may be described in three stages: 1) acute and immediate effects, 2) intermediate effects, and 3) long-term reactions.

Acute and Immediate Effects

The acute and immediate symptoms following the death of a loved one are usually shock, disbelief, tearfulness, and a sense of unreality, combined with a spectrum of emotions such as sadness, fear, anger, helplessness, and anxiety. Children's grief responses are associated not only with sadness but also with somatic symptoms, changes in behavior, social withdrawal, decreased interest in previously enjoyed activities, regressive behaviors, irritability, and decrements in school performance. Children may become preoccupied with their own fears of death. Each child has to struggle to adjust to changing life circumstances, to resume normal activities, and to begin the process of investing in new relationships, and yet maintain an appropriate attachment to the lost loved one through reminiscences and memorabilia.

Often, soon after the death of a loved one, children experience loss of appetite, sleep disturbances, and aching pain in the pit of the stomach. Bereavement is accompanied by disturbances in thinking, such as decreased concentration, diminished capacity for problem solving, and inability to think about consequences or plan for the future. Younger children may manifest regression, agitation, disorganized behaviors, clinging dependency, bodily symptoms, loss of bladder or bowel control, and nightmares. Children may experience preoccupation with death, health issues, altered perceptions (e.g., seeing the lost person on the street), and vivid dreams of the deceased.

Kranzler et al. (1990) studied preschool children, ages 3–6 years, who had lost a parent. Compared with nonbereaved children, children who had lost a parent were more scared and unhappy, and experienced significantly more emotional and behavioral symptoms. In contrast to responses of adults, children's grief responses were more episodic and situational but less pervasive. Other researchers have noted that children often manifest less sadness and emotional turmoil than adults in the immediate aftermath of the loss of a loved one. In a study of children ages 5–12 years conducted 3 months after the death of a parent, the following rates of bereavement symptoms were observed: loss of appetite (24%), depressed mood (61%), loss of interest (45%), feelings of guilt/worthlessness (37%), sleep disturbances (32%), and suicidal ideation (61%) (Weller et al. 1991). The suicidal ideation represented a longing to be with the deceased parent (reunion fantasy) rather than the devaluation of the child's own life, and none of the children attempted suicide.

Intermediate Effects

The intermediate effects of bereavement for children may include ongoing difficulties in social relatedness including social withdrawal, somatic symptoms, waves of distress, a preoccupation with the image of the departed, yearning for the deceased, impaired vocational and school adjustment, nightmares, loss of appetite, weight loss, sleep disturbances, suicidal thoughts, loss of interest in normally enjoyed activities, a limited range of emotions or excessive emotionality, and clinging-dependent regressive behaviors. Depending on their level of cognitive development, children may want explanations as to the cause of what happened and may search for blame. Not understanding cause-and-effect reactions, young children may blame themselves for the death. Children may neglect self-care, fail to perform household chores, or experience a decline in academic or work performance. Children may demonstrate angry, aggressive, and antisocial behaviors, in addition to a spectrum of anxiety and depressive symptoms.

Long-Term Reactions

Children may experience long-term reactions to bereavement, which include further decrements in academic performance; a range of anxiety, depressive, and behavioral symptoms; bodily symptoms; interpersonal and social adjustment problems; and decreased self-efficacy. Worden and Silverman (1996) studied 125 children who had experienced the death of a parent. Compared with matched control subjects, bereaved children were more likely to exhibit lower self-esteem and lower scores on locus of control. Approximately one-fifth of the bereaved children manifested serious emotional and behavioral disturbances requiring intervention. Two years after the parental death, preadolescent girls were more prone to experience anxiety, depression, and aggressive behaviors, whereas adolescent boys were more socially withdrawn and exhibited more social problems.

Prolonged Grief Reactions

Increasing interest has been shown in what has been defined as a *prolonged grief disorder* or *chronic mourning*. Individuals with prolonged grief reactions are preoccupied with intense yearning for the deceased, continuing intrusive thoughts about the deceased, feelings of anger, emotional numbness, and a sense of hopelessness with some functional impairment (Lichtenthal et al. 2004). The sudden, often horrific, unexpected death of a loved one—an event frequently associated with disaster—is a risk factor for prolonged grief (Maguen et al. 2009). A survey of 704 bereaved adults 3–5 years after the September 11 attacks found that 43% met criteria for prolonged grief, which was often comorbid with PTSD and depression (Neria et al. 2007).

Childhood Bereavement and Psychological Morbidity

Adults identified as having experienced maternal death before age 10 were observed to have increased risks for panic attacks and simple phobias in later life (Tweed et al. 1989). Breier et al. (1988) noted that a child who experiences the early death of a parent is at increased risk for psychiatric disorders (particularly depression) in adult life, although the risk is diminished for the bereaved child who maintains a good relationship with the surviving parent and experiences satisfying peer relationships. Studies of bereaved children who have experienced the sudden death of a parent have indicated that they experience more anxiety, depression, and disruptive behaviors than their nonbereaved counterparts (Kranzler et al. 1990; Van Eerdewegh et al. 1985; Weller et al. 1991; Worden and Silverman 1996). Gleser et al. (1981) noted that in the West Virginia Buffalo Creek flood disaster, bereavement and threat to life were the predominant stressors giving rise to prolonged psychopathology. In a study of children ages 5–12 years, conducted 3 months after the death of a parent, Weller et al. (1991) found that 37% met diagnostic criteria for major depressive disorder. Surviving parents were not fully aware of their children's depressive symptoms, a finding that underscores the importance of interviewing bereaved children and not relying solely on parents' reports of their children's symptoms.

A study of Israeli children ages 2–10 years, conducted for several years following the death of their fathers in war, found that more than half demonstrated fears, overdependent behavior, and temper tantrums (Elizur and Kaffman 1982, 1983). Forty percent had emotional and behavioral problems of such severity as to interfere with adjustment at home, in school, and with peers. The severity of the bereavement reactions was influenced by the quality of the relationship with the father prior to his death, the ability of the mother to share her grief with the child, and the availability of extended family members to offer support. Other studies confirm that the psychological impact of parental death is predominantly mediated by the availability of extended family support systems, the relationship to the remaining parent, and other social and economic adversities (Breier et al. 1988; Harrington and Harrison 1999). Protective factors that help buffer the impact of bereavement are high self-esteem, calm temperament, scholastic competence, and ability to use available social support networks (Harrington and Harrison 1999). Table 6–3 indicates some of the risk factors associated with sustained bereavement.

Treatment Strategies

Usually, adults have the task of informing a child of the death of a family member, providing some explanation commensurate with the child's level of understanding, and ascribing meaning to the death in line with the family's religious beliefs. Death should not be likened to sleep or a long journey, but rather should be explained in terms of cessation of bodily activities. A number of children's books (e.g., *Charlotte's Web*, by

TABLE 6–3.	Factors in determining children's vulnerability to sustained bereavement

Perceived importance of relationship

Quality of relationship to deceased

Sudden and unexpected death

Circumstances of death

Cognitive maturity of child

Not having chance to say good-bye

Quality of family and social supports

Child's specific coping and adaptive skills

Socioeconomic supports

E. B. White) are useful for helping children to understand death as a natural phenomenon. Such readings increase awareness that exposure to death is part of the life experience.

Because grief is the normal psychological response to the death of a loved one, providers must be judicious in prescribing treatment interventions. They may have difficulty, however, distinguishing between a normal grief reaction and one that evolves with symptoms of depression and anxiety that interfere with the child's normal development and ability to meet the demands of everyday life. Depressive symptoms and suicidal thoughts are not uncommon. Caretakers and professionals should be aware of the potential for significant behavioral problems, emotional distress, bodily symptoms, declines in school performance, or impairment in interpersonal and social relationships for grieving children.

Making a Referral

A referral to mental health professionals should be considered when there is increasing concern about the child's ability to meet ordinary, everyday expectations. Indicators for treatment following bereavement may include a history of previous emotional or behavioral problems or current depressive, anxiety, and behavioral symptoms that interfere with the child's progressive development. Usually, a child is not identified as having significant emotional or behavioral problems until 6–12 months after the loss. Treatment goals should focus on providing a safe place, facilitating the acceptance of death, supporting new attachments and adjustments, restoring normal development, resolving mixed feelings, examining both positive and negative memories, clarifying cognitive distortions, and identifying mood states and traumatic reminders. Providers must distinguish between the psychological effects associated with posttraumatic stress responses and those associated with bereavement.

Some of the clues suggesting need for referral of a child are sustained poor academic performance, enduring distress, increasing social isolation, persistent mood dysregulation manifested by irritability, hyperarousal, expressed suicidal ideation such as a wish to join the departed, and/or evidence of depression with self-recrimination and guilt as if the child felt responsible for the death of the loved one.

Therapeutic interventions for bereaved children range from acute crisis intervention and brief psychosocial intervention to more intensive cognitive-behavioral therapies, psychodynamic/play therapies, and family and group therapy approaches.

Psychosocial and Crisis Intervention

Psychosocial and crisis intervention focuses on mobilizing family and social supports, encouraging positive adaptive and coping strategies, providing psychoeducation about expectable reactions that may be experienced, providing outlets for expression of feelings, reframing distorted thinking, and applying anxiety reduction techniques. The therapist stresses that the psychological response is a normally expected reaction to loss. The bereaved child is encouraged to restore routines; engage in health-promoting activities; and participate in social relationships, as well as normal school and work activities.

Cognitive-Behavioral Therapies

Trauma-focused cognitive-behavioral therapy (TF-CBT) is well established as an effective treatment for PTSD, anxiety, and depressive symptoms (Pine and Cohen 2002). TF-CBT encompasses many techniques, such as cognitive restructuring, exposure techniques, and emotional/information processing strategies. Cognitive restructuring explores the child's thoughts about a traumatic event with the goal of correcting inaccurate thinking or "cognitive distortions" (Pine and Cohen 2002). Young children not infrequently experience feelings of blame and guilt for the death of a loved one, or other inappropriate attributions for traumatic events. Through TF-CBT, children learn to examine their thoughts more critically, to avoid overgeneralizing, and to selectively attend to thoughts that are more accurate and helpful. Exposure techniques are often a part of CBT; these include reliving memories, writing personal narratives of the trauma, and maintaining a journal. The guided exposure provides a means by which the child can gradually absorb a traumatic experience over time. These strategies provide opportunities to confront traumatic reminders, which help to reduce the child's negative emotions, cognitive distortions, damaged self-efficacy, and feelings of guilt, anger, and helplessness. Therapeutic activities incorporate relaxation training and use of psychoeducational materials.

Cohen et al. (2006b) developed a cognitive-behavioral intervention specifically for childhood traumatic grief (CBT-CTG). The trauma-focused components include sessions on improving affect modulation, stress reduction, trauma-specific exposure, preserving positive memories, and defining the meaning of the loss. Cohen et al. (2006a) employed a modified 12-session version of their intervention with a sample of 39 children, ages 6–17 years, who were referred to outpatient treatment for child trauma and traumatic grief. Children showed significant improvement in grief, traumatic grief, mood, anxiety, posttraumatic stress, and behavior. An online training curriculum is available for CBT-CTG on CTG Web (http://ctg.musc.edu) for those who have completed the TF-CBT Web course (http://tfcbt.musc.edu).

Play Therapy

Play therapy relies on children's natural propensity to express their innermost conflicts in the symbolic world of play. Children attempt to solve problems through play. Play involves wish fulfillment and facilitates expression of pent-up feelings. In play therapy, children replace passivity with action and achieve mastery through experimentation and trial action. The child moves at his or her own pace with the therapist's clarifications and interventions. The therapist helps the child to understand and give meaning to grief and assists the child in restoring normal, age-appropriate developmental progression and adaptive coping strategies.

Family and Group Interventions

TF-CBT interventions may include a parent component that parallels the child's intervention, with the goal of enhancing parent-child communication as a part of the child's treatment (Pine and Cohen 2002). Black and Urbanowicz (1987) developed a six-session family intervention for children who had lost a parent before age 16 years, which focused on facilitating mourning for both the bereaved child and the surviving parent. Compared with the control group (24 families) at 1-year follow-up, the

---

TABLE 6–4.   Recommendations for parents to help their child deal with death

---

- *Meet as a family.* Provide a sense of a family working together to plan for the changes in family circumstances. The best support against loss is the love and support of other family members. Be sure to include the child as much as possible in family decisions.

- *Reassure the child.* Be a calm presence as much as possible. Let the child know the family is planning on how to stay together.

- *Recognize that children are children.* Children at different ages have different ideas about death. Help them to understand the meaning of death in its finality but in line with the family's religious beliefs.

- *Talk to your child in language that he or she can understand.* Explain to your child what happened, what is happening, and what is going to happen in a language that he or she can understand.

- *Listen to your child's feelings.* Younger children may not be able to express their grief, fears, and anxieties. It is often helpful to label the feelings and to validate them in a sensitive, supportive, and shared manner. Where possible, join with your child in understanding his or her feelings in a way that conveys that you will manage the situation. Allow your child to mourn or grieve.

- *Listen to your child's thoughts.* Try to understand your child's perceptions and thoughts about what has happened. Be aware of a readiness for self-blame, anger, and guilt. Listen and answer his or her questions honestly.

- *Encourage your child to talk.* Provide an atmosphere of acceptance in which the child feels free to express anxieties, grief, fears, and worries.

- *Routinize and normalize your child's life.* Get back to a routine as quickly as possible. This indicates to your child that you feel secure and are beginning to manage the situation.

---

treatment group (21 families) showed a trend toward more positive outcomes in mood, health, and behavior. Salloum et al. (2001), using a 10-session community-based grief and trauma group for adolescents ages 11–19 years who had lost a family member to homicide, found significant reductions in posttraumatic stress symptoms, specifically in reexperiencing and avoidance symptoms.

Parents can benefit from advice about helping their children deal with grief. See Table 6–4 for examples of recommendations that may be given to parents.

Attending the Funeral

Therapists are often asked whether children should attend funerals. Although the literature is contradictory and anecdotal on this point, therapists generally concur that if children are under age 5–6 years, they cannot process the meaning or understand the significance of what transpires. Increasing evidence does suggest, however, that when children want to go to a funeral, it may be psychologically beneficial if they are adequately prepared, informed, and accompanied by an adult who can be emotionally and cognitively available to comfort them and to manage any distress or grief occurring during the service. Participation in the funeral service may help children to remember loved ones and may provide an opportunity to say good-bye.

■ Key Clinical Points

- Children exposed to disaster may experience the death of a parent or other significant persons in their lives.

- Child traumatic grief differs from normal bereavement in that the former is a convergence of loss through death and traumatic exposure.

- A child's psychological reactions to the death of a loved one are influenced by the child's age, level of psychological and emotional maturity, extent of adaptive and coping capacities, and understanding of death.

- A child's responses to death are shaped by the child's relationship to the deceased, the circumstances of death, the child's previous experience with death, and available social support systems.

- Children's psychological reactions to death can be understood as evolving over time with acute, intermediate, and long-term consequences.

- The majority of bereaved children do not develop psychiatric disorders.

- Multiple and diverse intervention strategies can be attempted.

- Trauma-focused cognitive-behavioral therapy has the most empirical evidence demonstrating efficacy.

References

Black D, Urbanowicz MA: Family intervention with bereaved children. J Child Psychol Psychiatry 28:467–476, 1987

Breier A, Kelsoe JR, Kirwin PD, et al: Early parental loss and development of adult psychopathology. Arch Gen Psychiatry 45:987–993, 1988

Breslau N, Kessler RC, Chilcoat HD, et al: Trauma and posttraumatic stress disorder in the community: the 1996 Detroit Area Survey of Trauma. Arch Gen Psychiatry 55:626–632, 1998

Cohen JA, Mannarino AP, Gibson LE, et al: Interventions for children and adolescents following disaster, in Interventions Following Mass Violence and Disasters. Edited by Ritchie EC, Watson PJ, Friedman MJ. New York, Guilford, 2006a, pp 227–256

Cohen JA, Mannarino AP, Staron VR: A pilot study of modified cognitive behavioral therapy for childhood traumatic grief. J Am Acad Child Adolesc Psychiatry 45:1465–1473, 2006b

Dowdney L: Annotation: childhood bereavement following parental death. J Child Psychol Psychiatry 41:819–830, 2000

Elizur E, Kaffman M: Children's bereavement reactions following death of the father. J Am Acad Child Adolesc Psychiatry 21:474–480, 1982

Elizur E, Kaffman M: Factors influencing the severity of childhood bereavement reactions. Am J Orthopsychiatry 53:668–676, 1983

Gleser GC, Green B, Winget C: Prolonged Psychological Effects of Disaster: A Study of Buffalo Creek. New York, Academic Press, 1981

Harrington R, Harrison L: Unproven assumptions about the impact of bereavement on children. J R Soc Med 99:230–233, 1999

Kranzler EM, Shaffer D, Wasserman G, et al: Early childhood bereavement. J Am Acad Child Adolesc Psychiatry 29:513–520, 1990

Lichtenthal WG, Cruess DG, Prigerson HG: A case for establishing complicated grief as a distinct mental disorder in DSM-V. Clin Psychol Rev 24:637–662, 2004

Maguen A, Neria Y, Conocscenti L, et al: Depression and prolonged grief in the wake of disaster, in Mental Health and Disaster. Edited by Neria Y, Galea S, Norris FH. Cambridge, UK, Cambridge University Press, 2009, pp 116–130

National Center for Health Statistics: National Summary of Injury Mortality Data. Atlanta, GA, National Center for Injury and Prevention and Control, 1997

Neria Y, Gross R, Litz, B, et al: Prevalence and psychological correlates of complicated grief among bereaved adults 2.5–5 years after September 11th attacks. J Trauma Stress 20:251–262, 2007

Pfefferbaum B, North CS, Doughty DE, et al: Trauma, grief, and depression in Nairobi children after the 1998 bombing of the American Embassy. Death Stud 30:561–577, 2006

Pine OS, Cohen JA: Trauma in children and adolescents: risk and treatment of psychiatric sequelae. Biol Psychiatry 51:519–531, 2002

Prigerson HG, Bierhals AJ, Stanislav V, et al: Traumatic grief as a risk factor for mental and physical morbidity. Am J Psychiatry 154:616–623, 1997

Pynoos RS, Nader K, Frederick C, et al: Grief reactions in school age children following a sniper attack at school. Isr J Psychiatry Relat Sci 24:53–63, 1987

Raphael B: Grieving the death of a child. BMJ 332:620–621, 2006

Salloum A, Avery L, McClain RP: Group psychotherapy for adolescent survivors of homicide victims: a pilot study. J Am Acad Child Adolesc Psychiatry 40:1261–1267, 2001

Spence MW, Brent SB: Children's understanding of death: a review of three components of a death concept. Child Dev 55:1671–1686, 1984

Tweed JL, Schoenback VJ, George LK, et al: The effects of childhood parental death and divorce on six-month history of anxiety disorders. Br J Psychiatry 154:823–828, 1989

Van Eerdewegh, Clayton PJ, Van Eerdewegh P, et al: The bereaved child: variables influencing early psychopathology. Br J Psychiatry 147:188–194, 1985

Weller RA, Weller EB, Fristad MA, et al: Depression in recently bereaved prepubertal children. Am J Psychiatry 148:1536–1540, 1991

Wickrama KA, Kaspar V: Family context of mental health risk in tsunami-exposed adolescents: findings from a pilot study in Sri Lanka. Soc Sci Med 64:713–723, 2007

Worden JW, Silverman PR: Parental death and the adjustment of school-age children. Omega 33:91–102, 1996

Child and Family Assessment

Introduction

Disasters and traumatic events confront children and adults with a variety of stressors during the impact phase and in the aftermath. Assessment of the child and his or her family or caregivers is critical to determine the full extent of the child's psychological responses to life-threatening events.

The awareness that children encounter the same constellation of stressors as adults has increased the focus on evaluation of children exposed to traumatic events. Careful assessment of children's psychological reactions is essential for identifying children at elevated risk for disaster-related psychosocial consequences and children in need of therapeutic intervention, as well as for accurately diagnosing trauma-related symptoms. Despite the natural inclination to focus exclusively on posttraumatic stress symptoms, clinicians need to remember the spectrum of internalizing, externalizing, and somatic symptoms that children may experience as a result of the associated losses and the secondary adversities that occur in the aftermath of disaster.

In many instances, children will have preexisting psychiatric disorders that will confound the clinical presentation and will require a careful assessment to discern the many contributing elements to the clinical presentation. In choosing assessment strategies, clinicians need to stay attuned to possible coexisting psychological morbidities, such as mood disorder, other anxiety disorder, somatic ills, and behavioral problems.

Screening

Screening and evaluation of children and their families are conducted in a phase-specific manner over time. Informal assessment occurs on an ongoing basis as first responders, school personnel, and public health professionals interact with children and families who have been exposed to disaster. First responders begin the process of identifying children at high risk.

Those who are screening children and their families must be familiar with the spectrum of postdisaster psychological sequelae and be able to ask specific questions to elicit relevant psychological responses. Clinicians need to be sensitive to the child's level of cognitive and emotional development and obtain information from multiple sources, including the child, parents, and other caretakers.

More systematic approaches to screening may be implemented when the child has the opportunity to meet with crisis intervention specialists, school personnel, and other mental health professionals. Screening procedures are often administered in the school setting to help identify at-risk children and to facilitate appropriate interventions when indicated on behalf of these children and their families. Initial screening is focused on posttraumatic stress symptoms, whereas instruments for screening for other psychological morbidities are usually reserved for a later date, often when the child is in school or when referred to mental health professionals.

Standard Screening Instruments for Posttraumatic Stress Symptoms

Two self-report instruments that have been used rather commonly for posttraumatic stress symptoms are the Child PTSD Symptom Scale (CPSS; Foa et al. 2001) and the UCLA Posttraumatic Stress Disorder

Reaction Index (UCLA PTSD RI). The CPSS is a 24-item problem list that can be completed in approximately 15 minutes and may be administered individually or in a group format. The UCLA PTSD RI screening instrument is available in five versions: child, adolescent, parent, and abbreviated child and parent forms (Cohen et al. 2008; Steinberg et al. 2004). The child and adolescent versions (comprising 20 and 22 items, respectively) can be administered in an interview format or in a school classroom. The parent form has 21 items and is used to assess the younger child. (Information on availability of these instruments is supplied in Table 7–3, later in chapter.)

Brief Parent Screening Instruments

Parents or caretakers are usually asked to complete screening instruments for children younger than 8 years. The 21-item Pediatric Emotional Distress Scale (PEDS; Saylor et al. 1999) is useful as a brief screening instrument for parents to report emotional distress in children ages 2–10 years after exposure to a stressful or traumatic event. (Information on availability is supplied in Table 7–3, later in chapter.) The 6-item Brief Parent Screening Version of the UCLA PTSD RI has been developed to be completed by parents of children younger than 8 years (Cohen et al. 2008). The form is shown in Figure 7–1.

Brief Child Screening Instruments

Children older than 7 years are usually able to self-report trauma exposure symptoms. A 9-item Abbreviated UCLA PTSD RI Child Version was developed for assessment and screening of students after the September 11, 2001, attacks on America and has been reported to have good sensitivity and specificity for detecting PTSD (Steinberg et al. 2004; see also Cohen et al. 2008). Children with a score of 10 or higher are thought to have clinically significant PTSD symptoms (Cohen et al. 2008). The abbreviated self-report version is shown in Figure 7–2 (Cohen et al. 2008; Pynoos and Steinberg 2001).

Screening will indicate, in some instances, that children and their families need to be referred to a mental health professional for a more formal evaluation. Referrals are warranted for symptoms and behaviors that are severe and hinder the child's ability to meet the demands of everyday life. For the younger child, indicators may include excessive and persistent fearfulness, clinging and dependent behaviors, temper tantrums, agitation, hyperactivity, loss of bladder and bowel control, and disturbing

Instructions to parent: You have said that something really scary or upsetting has happened to your child or family. Please circle how often your child has had the following problems related to that, IN THE PAST MONTH.

	Hardly ever	Sometimes	A lot
1. When something reminds my child of what happened he or she gets very upset, scared, or sad.	0	1	2
2. My child has upsetting thoughts, pictures, or sounds of what happened come into his or her mind when he or she does not want them to.	0	1	2
3. My child feels grouchy, angry, or mad.	0	1	2
4. My child tries to stay away from people, places, or things that make him or her remember what happened.	0	1	2
5. My child is more aggressive (hitting, biting, kicking, or breaking things) since this happened.	0	1	2
6. My child has trouble going to sleep or wakes up often during the night.	0	1	2

FIGURE 7–1.   Abbreviated UCLA Posttraumatic Stress Disorder Reaction Index (PTSD RI) Parent Version.

Source.   Cohen et al. 2008. Copyright 2008, Robert S. Pynoos, M.D., Alan M. Steinberg, Ph.D., and Michael S. Scheeringa, M.D. Used with permission.

Here is a list of nine problems people sometimes have after very bad things happen. Think about your traumatic experience and circle one of the numbers (0, 1, 2, 3, 4) that tells how often the problem happened to you DURING THE PAST MONTH. For example, 0 means not at all and 4 means almost every day.

	None	Little	Some	Much	Most
1. I get upset, afraid or sad when something makes me think about what happened.	❑ 0	❑ 1	❑ 2	❑ 3	❑ 4
2. I have upsetting thoughts or pictures of what happened come into my mind when I do not want them to.	❑ 0	❑ 1	❑ 2	❑ 3	❑ 4
3. I feel grouchy, or I am easily angered.	❑ 0	❑ 1	❑ 2	❑ 3	❑ 4
4. I try not to talk about, think about, or have feelings about what happened.	❑ 0	❑ 1	❑ 2	❑ 3	❑ 4
5. I have trouble going to sleep, or wake up often during the night.	❑ 0	❑ 1	❑ 2	❑ 3	❑ 4
6. I have trouble concentrating or paying attention.	❑ 0	❑ 1	❑ 2	❑ 3	❑ 4
7. I try to stay away from people, places, or things that make me remember what happened.	❑ 0	❑ 1	❑ 2	❑ 3	❑ 4
8. I have bad dreams, including dreams about what happened.	❑ 0	❑ 1	❑ 2	❑ 3	❑ 4
9. I feel alone inside and not close to other people.	❑ 0	❑ 1	❑ 2	❑ 3	❑ 4

FIGURE 7–2. Abbreviated UCLA Posttraumatic Stress Disorder Reaction Index (PTSD RI) for DSM-IV Child Version.

Source. Cohen et al. 2008. Copyright 2008, Robert S. Pynoos, M.D., Alan M. Steinberg, Ph.D., and Michael S. Scheeringa, M.D. Used with permission.

nightmares. For the older child or adolescent, symptoms of concern include hyperarousal, anxiety, panic, depressed mood, and such maladaptive behaviors as belligerence, family and interpersonal conflicts, decrease in academic performance, and misuse of substances.

Clinical Assessment

The clinician should take a careful assessment and clinical history from a child's parents or caretakers. Before children and parents are engaged in a psychological interview, safeguards should be in place to ensure that the child and family members are safe and secure, that life-sustaining provisions are assured, and that measures have been taken to provide continuity of support systems.

The clinical evaluation process is complex and multifaceted. It requires not only an interview with the child but also information from other informants, such as parents, family members, teachers, and other significant persons in the child's life. Because the family system may either hinder or facilitate the child's psychological adaptation and coping strategies, the clinician needs to evaluate the effects of disaster on the various members of the family, with particular focus on the parental response. Clinicians generally agree that family and parental support mitigates a child's risk for posttraumatic stress symptoms.

The parent interview elicits objective information regarding the nature and severity of the trauma exposure, stressors encountered, psychological responses (including possible posttraumatic stress symptoms), behavior problems, mood and anxiety symptoms, multiple unexplained physical symptoms, and concurrent psychological disorders. The parent interview explores the child's developmental history; risk and protective factors; parent and family responses to the disaster; and the ethnic, religious, and cultural context of the traumatic event. Table 7–1 lists the critical elements to be elicited in the assessment process.

In a separate interview, children are provided an opportunity to describe their perceptions and understanding of what happened and their reactions to the traumatic experience. The child interview should focus on engagement strategies, friendly interaction, empathic listening, and sensitivity to the child's emotional state and cognitive level. The use of nonverbal modalities such as play, storytelling, or drawings, as well as some direct questioning, is necessary to elicit the child's perception, understanding, and response to the traumatic situation.

The clinician needs to establish a sense of ease with the child, to slowly win the child's confidence through friendly interactions, and to find the child's level of discourse. In most instances, children are able to tell their stories in words or use nonverbal means for relating what happened as expressed in play, storytelling, and drawings. School-age children are usually able to provide self-reports of their traumatic exposures. Direct questioning is often necessary to fill in the gaps, but the questions should be sensitive to the child's comfort, emotional availability, and cognitive development. In Table 7–2, we list questions to ask the child during the interview.

Child assessment requires collecting information regarding the child's perceptions and understanding, theory of causality, self-attributions, resilience, and repertoire of adaptive and coping mechanisms for regulating emotions and impulse control. While gathering information through the parent and child interviews, the clinician should be aware of how the child's level of cognitive and emotional development influences the expression of posttraumatic stress symptoms. Because of their cognitive and emotional immaturity, children are often unable to fully discuss their distress and impairment. Infants and toddlers are limited in their expressive language skills and capabilities for describing their subjective experiences. Preschool children are unable to verbalize symptoms of distress, describe intrusive thoughts or flashbacks, or identify sources of physical complaints. For preschool children, internal emotional states are revealed through behaviors such as clinging and dependency, temper tantrums, separation anxiety, fear of the dark, and sleep and appetite disturbances (Scheeringa et al. 1995).

Piaget (1967) observed that younger children do not recognize the existence of chance happenings. The younger child assumes that everything that happens is related to something that he or she did or did not do. Before age 7 years, children often attribute purpose or intention to events that others realize are chance happenings.

For school-age children, the focus shifts to assessment of behavioral expressions of inner turmoil. Psychological distress may manifest through play and behavioral symptoms rather than through verbal description. Hyperactivity, sleep and appetite disturbances, decrements in school performance, inability to concentrate, physical symptoms, irritability, and sibling rivalry are common responses to the traumatic situation. In contrast, older children are often able to express unpleasant internal emotional states in words, discuss the subjective experience of the trauma exposure, and ascribe meaning to the event.

TABLE 7–1. Critical elements elicited in the child and family posttrauma assessment process

History of the traumatic exposure

Assess the traumatic event as an extreme stressor
  What is the nature of the traumatic event?
Does it qualify as an imagined or actual threat to bodily integrity or to life itself?
What was the level of exposure?
  Direct physical impact, visual or media exposure, interpersonal relatedness to victims
  What was the intensity and duration of exposure?

Family history

Were the parents and other family members exposed?
What was the parental or family response to the traumatic event?
Elicit information regarding:
  Parents' emotional and behavioral symptoms
  Parents' psychopathology
  Parents' reaction to the child's distress
  Family mental health history
  Stability and functionality of the family support system
  Ethnic/cultural history

Inventory of stressors

Evaluate presence and extent of the following:
  Bereavement
  Separation from loved ones
  Loss of home/shelter
  Loss of school or other routine activities
  Relationship to peer group
  Physical injury

Child's developmental history

Assess the following:
  Previous exposure to traumatic events
  Coping behaviors
  Psychosocial adjustment
  Psychological morbidity
  History of psychological treatments
  Medical history
  School and academic performance

TABLE 7–1.   Critical elements elicited in the child and family posttrauma assessment process (*continued*)

Child interview

Obtain child's report of what happened

Explore child's attributions and understanding of:

  What happened

  Why it happened

  Thoughts and feelings about what happened

  His or her self-perceived role in what happened

  How the trauma has affected his or her emotional and
    behavioral well-being

Complete a symptom inventory

Assess for acute stress disorder and
  posttraumatic stress disorder

Assess for psychiatric comorbidity

  Mood disorder

  Anxiety disorder

  Adjustment disorders

  Disruptive behaviors: attention-deficit/hyperactivity disorder,
    conduct disorder, oppositional defiant disorder

  Symptoms of hyperarousal

  Substance abuse

  Dissociative disorders

  Physical symptoms

Assess self-efficacy, coping, and adaptive capacities

Assess child's capacities to seek and use help from adults

TABLE 7–2.   The child interview: direct questions to consider

---

Have you been hurt or injured?

Have you seen anyone get hurt badly?

Has anyone in your family been hurt?

Have you seen anything really scary and frightening?

Do you ever have any scary dreams or nightmares?

How do you sleep at night?

What was the most upsetting and scary part of the experience?

Do you ever see or hear anything that reminds you of something really scary?

Who makes you feel safe?

Source.   Adapted from Bostic and King 2007.

PTSD Rating Scales and Instruments

The ability to understand the clinical ramifications of the impact of disaster on children and families has been strengthened by the development of formal psychometric instruments to screen and assess psychological reactions (Saylor and Deroma 2002). Standardized instruments for the assessment of posttraumatic stress symptoms and the broader range of psychological reactions are often useful. Standardized assessment instruments target specific dimensions of disaster or trauma exposure and help to identify stressors, emotional and behavioral reactions, and attributions of causation. Optimal assessment includes the use of multiple information sources and the selection of well-established, reliable, and valid assessment measures (Finch and Daugherty 1993).

To properly select an assessment approach, the clinician must clarify the goals and define the key questions for investigation. One primary question is whether the assessment will be used for triage purposes or as a tool to define the child's psychological responses to the traumatic event. Assessment procedures may be used as part of a triage process to identify children at high risk, to identify children with emotional and behavioral problems that interfere with their ability to meet the demands of everyday life, or to identify children with psychiatric disorders such as PTSD or depression.

Balaban (2006) identified five field-tested screening instruments designed for children and adolescents that are applicable for use in disaster and emergency settings. Each instrument employs a standardized, scientifically validated questionnaire that can be administered by clinicians or nonclinicians in 60 minutes or less. Balaban concluded that of the five measures, the UCLA PTSD RI is the most appropriate measure for evaluating children across a wide variety of disasters. This measure, now available in multiple languages, is inexpensive, simple, rapidly administered and scored, and supported by sound scientific research. Instruments commonly used for assessing posttraumatic symptoms and PTSD are described in Table 7–3.

Rating Scales for Coexisting Psychological Morbidities

In addition to posttraumatic stress symptoms, mood and anxiety symptoms are common responses to the life-threatening situations and multiple losses that characterize disasters. Standardized instruments for the broader range of psychological and behavioral reactions are briefly described in Table 7–4.

■ Key Clinical Points

- The assessment of the child and family is critical for determining the full extent of the child's psychological responses to life-threatening events.
- Children who are judged to be at high risk of stress symptoms following disaster or a traumatic event should be identified for screening.
- Screening instruments are available for eliciting trauma-related symptoms.
- The child should be interviewed individually when possible.
- The assessment process must be sensitive to the child's level of cognitive and emotional development.
- Optimal assessment uses multiple sources of information to provide understanding of the child's psychological responses.
- Assessing the postdisaster psychosocial functioning of the family is essential.
- Specific psychometric measures can be employed to assess trauma-related symptoms as well as coexisting psychological morbidities.

TABLE 7–3.   Instruments for assessing posttraumatic symptoms and PTSD

Instrument	Purpose	Availability	Ages (years)	Length/ administration time
UCLA PTSD Reaction Index for DSM-IV	To assess posttrauma symptoms and PTSD in children	No cost; see http://www.ptsd.va.gov/ professional/pages/assessments/ ucla-ptsd-dsm-iv.asp	6–17	20–22 items 20–30 minutes
Impact of Events Scale—Revised (IES-R)	To measure symptoms of PTSD after a traumatic event	No cost; available on many Web sites A 13-item version (IES-13) developed for children affected by war is available at www.childrenandwar.org/measures	Not designed for children, but used with children as young as 7	22 items 10–15 minutes
Child PTSD Symptom Scale (CPSS)	To evaluate symptoms and functional impairment related to PTSD	No cost; see http://www.ptsd.va.gov/ professional/pages/assessments/ cpss.asp	8–18	24 items 15 minutes
Posttraumatic Stress Symptoms in Children (PTSS-C)	To identify pediatric posttraumatic symptoms in chaotic disaster contexts	No cost	6–18	30 items 30 minutes
Trauma Symptom Checklist for Children (TSCC)	To assess PTSD symptoms after trauma, particularly sexual abuse	Licensed through www.parinc.com	7–16	54 items 20 minutes

Note.   PTSD=posttraumatic stress disorder.
Source.   Adapted from Balaban 2006.

TABLE 7–4. Rating scales for coexisting psychological morbidities

Instrument	Purpose	Availability	Ages (years)	Length/administration time
Depression scales				
Children's Depression Inventory 2 (CDI 2)	To measure depressive symptom severity in children	Licensed through www.mhs.com	7–17	28 items 5–15 minutes
Birleson Depression Self-Rating Scale (DSRS)	To measure symptoms of depression	No cost; contact author	6–13	18 items
Anxiety scales				
Multidimensional Anxiety Scale for Children (MASC)	To assess anxiety symptoms in children	Licensed through www.mhs.com	8–19	39 items[a] 15 minutes
Revised Children's Manifest Anxiety Scale, 2nd Edition (RCMAS-2)	To evaluate anxiety symptoms in children	Licensed through www.mhs.com	6–19	49 items 10–15 minutes
behavior scales				
atric Emotional Distress e (PEDS)	To measure posttraumatic behavioral problems in children	No cost; see www.nctsn.org	2–10	21 items 10–15 minutes
Behavior Problem st (RBPC)	To rate problem behavior in adolescents and young children	Licensed through www.parinc.com	5–18	89 items 20 minutes

ort form also available.
pted from Balaban 2006.

References

Balaban V: Psychological assessment of children in disasters and emergencies. Disasters 30:178–198, 2006

Bostic JQ, King RA: Clinical assessment of children and adolescents: content and structure, in Lewis's Child and Adolescent Psychiatry. Edited by Martin A, Volkmar FR. Philadelphia, PA, Wolters Kluwer, 2007, pp 323–344

Cohen JA, Kelleher KJ, Mannarino AP: Identifying, treating, and referring traumatized children: the role of pediatric providers. Arch Pediatr Adolesc Med 162:447–452, 2008

Finch AJ, Daugherty TK: Issues in the assessment of posttraumatic stress disorder in children, in Children and Disasters. Edited by Saylor CF. New York, Plenum Press, 1993, pp 45–66

Foa EB, Johnson KM, Feeny NC, et al: The Child PTSD Symptom Scale: a preliminary examination of its psychometric properties. J Clin Child Psychol 30:376–384, 2001

Piaget J: Six Psychological Studies. New York, Random House, 1967

Pynoos RS, Steinberg AM: Abbreviated UCLA PTSD Reaction Index for DSM-IV. Los Angeles, CA, National Center for Child Traumatic Stress, 2001

Saylor C, Deroma V: Assessment of children and adolescents exposed to disaster, in Helping Children Cope With Disasters and Terrorism. Edited by La Greca AM, Silverman WK, Vernberg EM, et al. Washington, DC, American Psychological Association, 2002, pp 35–53

Saylor CF, Swenson CC, Reynolds SS, et al: The Pediatric Emotional Distress Scale: a brief screening measure for young children exposed to traumatic events. J Clin Child Psychol 28:70–81, 1999

Scheeringa MS, Zeanah CH, Drell MJ, et al: Two approaches to the diagnosis of posttraumatic stress disorder in infancy and early childhood. J Am Acad Child Adolesc Psychiatry 34:191–200, 1995

Steinberg AM, Brymer MJ, Decker KB, et al: The University of California at Los Angles Post-traumatic Stress Disorder Reaction Index. Curr Psychiatry Rep 6:96–100, 2004

8

Interventions

On successful completion of this chapter, you should be able to:

- Understand the general intervention strategies for working with survivors of disasters.

- Identify the range of psychosocial interventions for disaster-related psychological morbidities.

- Describe the key principles of Psychological First Aid as an intervention in the early days and weeks after disaster.

- Describe the key principles of Skills for Psychological Recovery as an intervention in the intermediate phase of recovery.

- Recognize that psychological debriefing should be used with caution.

- Recognize the role of psychopharmacology with children and adolescents following disaster.

- Recognize the importance of systems of care after disaster.

- Recognize that school-based interventions have a role in postdisaster interventions.

- Understand the role of the federal response.

Introduction

As research on traumatized children and their families has increased, so has the level of thoughtfulness regarding psychosocial interventions to facilitate recovery (National Commission on Children and Disasters 2010). Some general strategies (Table 8–1) seem to cut across the various psychosocial interventions used in work with survivors.

TABLE 8–1.   General intervention strategies

Provide a sense of safety and security.

Connect the child with family and social supports.

Provide information and decrease uncertainty.

Provide opportunities for children to tell their stories.

Reconstruct the child's understanding of what occurred.

Determine the child's definition of the situation.

Identify and help correct cognitive distortions.

Assess the inventory of stressors the child is experiencing.

Assess for psychological and psychiatric disorders.

Promote and facilitate resilience.

Provide carefully guided and controlled reexposure to the trauma as appropriate.

Clarify themes of guilt, betrayal, revenge, helplessness, and excitement.

Assess the impact of the event on child development.

Work with changed attitudes toward self, others, and the future.

Work with the loss of cherished beliefs.

Promote assimilation and integration of the traumatic experience.

Identify traumatic reminders.

Facilitate tolerance for disaster-related thoughts, feelings, and moods.

Provide therapy for identified psychiatric disorders.

Facilitate the continued integrity of family and social support systems.

Promote adaptive coping.

Facilitate the restoration of normal developmental trajectories.

General Intervention Principles

Psychological interventions are sequenced across the disaster timeline, which may best be conceptualized as specific phases: 1) the impact phase, 2) the acute or immediate phase (days to weeks), 3) the intermediate phase (weeks to months), and 4) the longer, sustained recovery period. Efforts are continuously being made to design empirically based psychosocial interventions to fit the needs of survivors, their location, and the phase-specific stages that occur across the disaster timeline. Parents and other important family members or designated caretakers are always integral to the therapeutic intervention with children and are an important component in virtually all treatment modalities.

Interventions implemented during the immediate and intermediate postdisaster phases are designed to reduce distress and hyperarousal and to provide information. Two such interventions are Psychological First Aid (PFA) and Skills for Psychological Recovery (SPR). PFA is designed to be administered during the impact phase and in the early days and weeks after disaster, for the purpose of reducing distress and fear responses by providing a safe and secure environment, reducing uncertainty, mitigating fear and anxiety, and mobilizing family and social supports (National Child Traumatic Stress Network and National Center for PTSD [NCTSN and NCPTSD] 2006). SPR is an evidence-informed modular skills training intervention designed to be employed in the weeks and months after disaster when community rebuilding is occurring and survivors are exposed to various adversities, secondary stressors, and the ongoing process of adapting to life-changing circumstances associated with the aftermath of disaster (Berkowitz et al. 2010a).

PFA and SPR can be provided by a wide range of disaster response mental and health care professionals. Other interventions, such as cognitive-behavioral therapy (CBT), are more specifically designed for emotional and behavioral disorders that are more enduring and that begin to interfere with the child's capacity to meet the demands of daily life. Psychoeducation and psychopharmacology may be used at any point along the timeline.

Because disasters impact the individual child and have reverberating effects on the family and larger community, interventions must be tailored for application to the individual, the family, and the encompassing community.

Early Interventions

In this section, we describe interventions for the impact phase, the acute or immediate phase, and the intermediate phase.

Extrication

In the impact phase, first-line responders, search and rescue personnel, emergency medical service, police, and fire personnel are often available to facilitate rescue and provide immediate relief. Extrication has evolved into a fire services function in most of the country. In addition to having specialized technical training as well as search and rescue teams, fire services have more experience with building collapse and secondary hazards (e.g., floods, fires) than other organizations. Medical personnel are accustomed to providing care to trauma victims. When numerous survivors need care in a disaster situation, however, triage becomes necessary to allocate limited resources. Triage must occur at multiple levels, and patients must be reassessed during every step of the process.

Psychological First Aid

PFA, an evidence-informed early intervention for disaster survivors of all ages, can be applied in the immediate aftermath of disaster. It is a supportive intervention that is designed for delivery by mental health and other disaster response workers who provide early assistance to affected children, families, and adults as part of an organized disaster response effort. PFA is intended to reduce acute psychological distress, enhance resilience, and foster adaptive coping (NCTSN and NCPTSD 2006). The conceptual origins of PFA are diverse approaches to mitigating stress following trauma exposure, such as crisis intervention, military psychiatry, disaster psychiatry, and trauma psychiatry (Lindemann 1944; Mitchell 1983; Pynoos and Nader 1988; Ursano and Friedman 2006).

Following the September 11, 2001, attacks on America, the National Institute of Mental Health convened two expert consensus conferences to review the scientific research literature and to recommend a comprehensive approach to early intervention following mass trauma (National Institute of Mental Health 2002). The international expert panel recommended a multifaceted approach that specified PFA as one key component. Thereafter, federal funding was appropriated for the creation of a model PFA intervention. The outcome of this expert-driven endeavor was the development of *Psychological First Aid Field Operations Guide*, which is currently in its second edition (NCTSN and NCPTSD 2006). The two lead agencies that coordinated the development of PFA were the National Center for Child Traumatic Stress and the National Center for PTSD, thus ensuring the applicability of this intervention to children and adolescents as well as adults of all ages.

In the second edition of the *Psychological First Aid Field Operations Guide,* NCTSN and NCPTSD (2006) note,

> The principles and techniques of Psychological First Aid meet four basic standards. They are: (1) consistent with research evidence on risk and resilience following trauma; (2) applicable and practical in field settings; (3) appropriate for developmental levels across the lifespan; and (4) cul-

turally informed and adaptable. Psychological First Aid does not assume that all survivors will develop severe mental health problems or long-term difficulties in recovery, but instead is based on an understanding that disaster survivors and others affected by such events will experience a broad range of early reactions (for example physical, psychological, behavioral, spiritual). Some of these reactions will cause enough distress to interfere with adaptive coping, and may be mitigated by compassionate and caring disaster responders.

Thus, PFA is designed to foster adaptive functioning and coping for disaster survivors in the early days and weeks after disaster. An underlying assumption is that survivors have a natural impetus to recovery, and the task of rescue personnel is to facilitate that process and to restore psychological equilibrium. PFA attempts 1) to facilitate the family's natural resilience through reassurance, psychoeducation, encouragement for positive coping behaviors, and mobilization of family and social supports by linking survivors to available, practical resources; and 2) to mitigate distress and physiological arousal. PFA encourages survivors to take an active role in their recovery from disaster and to resume normal routines as quickly as possible. PFA providers reduce uncertainty by providing credible disaster event information regarding what has happened and what to expect.

PFA is premised on the fact that disaster survivors will experience a spectrum of psychological reactions. Whereas most will experience brief, transient distress, a smaller proportion may experience more enduring distress that interferes with adaptive functioning. PFA assumes that relatively few disaster survivors will progress to severe impairment or psychiatric illness. Most survivors will need no formal early intervention.

Survivors who are most likely to benefit from PFA are those with acute stress response symptoms and those with preexisting risk factors that increase vulnerability to the disaster or traumatic event. Although PFA may reduce distress in both adults and children, no evidence has shown that it will reduce the risk of subsequent psychological disorders. Participation is voluntary on the part of survivors. The basic objectives of PFA are noted in Table 8–2.

Reissman et al. (2006) suggested five essential tactical actions to enable the survivor to move forward to a more comfortable place psychologically in the immediate aftermath of disaster:

1. From risk to safety
2. From fear to calming
3. From loss to connectedness
4. From helplessness to efficacy
5. From despair to hopefulness

TABLE 8–2.	Basic objectives of Psychological First Aid

Establish a human connection in a nonintrusive and compassionate manner.

Enhance immediate and ongoing safety.

Provide physical and emotional comfort.

Calm and orient emotionally overwhelmed and distraught survivors.

Encourage survivors to express their needs and concerns.

Provide information and practical assistance.

Connect with family and social supports.

Facilitate positive coping strategies and resilience.

Link survivors with available services.

Source. National Child Traumatic Stress Network and National Center for PTSD 2006.

PFA providers are most effective when they approach disaster survivors with a calm, available, "compassionate presence." The initial tasks are to make contact with the child; provide life-sustaining safety, security, shelter, and sustenance (food, water, and clothing); and attend to basic comforts. A high priority is for PFA providers to facilitate the reuniting of the child with family members from whom they are separated. In their interactions with disaster-affected children, PFA providers will comfort, educate, listen supportively, and convey empathy and a sense of confidence that things are under control.

Some specific core actions (Table 8–3) may be employed to promote a child's and family's adaptive coping capacities. On the basis of the information gathered, the PFA provider selects and tailors one or more of these core actions to the individual survivor. The core actions include such activities as educating survivors about the effects of trauma and trauma reminders, normalizing and validating distress responses, and identifying available resources to aid recovery.

PFA providers need to observe and identify adults and children who are judged to be at elevated psychological risk and who may require more selective professional attention and support. Children at risk who might benefit from crisis intervention are those who manifest hyperarousal, intense anxiety, disorientation, psychological numbness, regressive behaviors, grief reactions, and dissociative responses. It is essential that providers identify the inventory of stressors each child has experienced and assess those children who have been physically injured, those who have had family members injured or killed, those who

---

TABLE 8–3.   Psychological First Aid core actions

---

1. Contact and engagement
2. Safety and comfort
3. Stabilization
4. Information gathering: current needs and concerns
5. Practical assistance
6. Connection with social supports
7. Information on coping
8. Linkage with collaborative services

Source.   National Child Traumatic Stress Network and National Center for PTSD 2006.

have been separated from loved ones, and those who lost their homes or valued personal possessions. Clinicians need to ascertain each child's current level of functioning, the predisaster level of functioning, and any incongruity in adaptation and coping skills to help decide whether further professional attention is indicated.

Crisis Intervention Strategies

A crisis involves an acute disruption of psychological equilibrium. A crisis is precipitated by exposure to a traumatic event coupled with the perception that this event is the cause of distress that is not easily resolved through the usual coping mechanisms. Crisis intervention is a strategy for reducing or eliminating specific symptoms with the intent of restoring disaster survivors to their precrisis level of functioning. Special attention should be given to extreme acute stress reactions, such as intense anxiety, depressed mood, anger, or hyperarousal, that interfere with coping; dissociative symptoms, such as derealization, depersonalization, and frozen emotionality; bodily symptoms; disturbed sleep; and impaired cognitive processing, including decreased concentration, confusion, and poor decision making (Young 2006).

Crisis intervention is a brief psychotherapy, usually presented in one to six sessions. Specific crisis intervention techniques include the use of relaxation exercises such as slow breathing, muscle relaxation, and guided imagery; cognitive reframing; and psychoeducation about expectable responses to trauma, positive and negative coping, and problem-solving strategies. Stress management approaches may include distraction techniques such as participating in social activities, play, or

---

TABLE 8–4.   Skills for Psychological Recovery: basic assumptions

---

Interventions must be

- Consistent with research evidence on risk and resilience.
- Applicable and practical in field setting.
- Appropriate for all developmental levels.
- Culturally informed.

Source.   Berkowitz et al. 2010a.

watching television. As much as possible, the mental health professional normalizes the child's psychological response to the traumatic event. In a supportive manner, the therapist allows the child to tell his or her story, but does not interrogate or press for responses. The therapist actively promotes recreation and physical activities such as exercise, sports, and dance; healthful diet and sleep patterns; social interactions with loved ones; and productive task or work experiences. The therapist also discourages the use of alcohol or drugs, social isolation, and excessive work. Crisis intervention has been shown to be efficacious in restoring predisaster functioning for both adults and youth (Auerbach and Kilmann 1977; Goenjian et al. 1997; Koss and Butcher 1986).

Skills for Psychological Recovery

SPR is a skills training intervention predicated on the recognition that in many instances, further psychosocial interventions will be required subsequent to the administration of PFA in the acute aftermath of disaster. NCTSN and NCPTSD developed SPR as a modular approach, to be used with disaster survivors to mitigate ongoing distress and to enhance coping with the cascade of postdisaster stressors (Berkowitz et al. 2010a). It is an evidence-informed modular intervention to help children, adolescents, adults, and their families to cope with the secondary adversities of disaster and the ongoing process of adapting to changing circumstances in their life experiences. According to the SPR developers, SPR is not a formal mental health treatment but rather an intervention designed to mitigate distress in the intermediate postdisaster phase of recovery. SPR as an intervention strategy is based on the assumptions noted in Table 8–4.

SPR is an intervention designed to reduce distress, identify coping skills, facilitate adaptation, and decrease the risk for emergent psychological morbidity and usually has a short duration (three to five sessions).

TABLE 8–5.   Skills for Psychological Recovery: goals and objectives

---

Protect the mental health of disaster survivors.

Enhance survivors' ability to address their concerns and needs.

Teach skills to promote the recovery of children, adolescents, adults, and families.

Prevent maladaptive behaviors while identifying and supporting adaptive behaviors.

Source.   Berkowitz et al. 2010a.

However, Berkowitz et al. (2010a) suggest that SPR can be delivered as a single stand-alone session. The stated goals and objectives are noted in Table 8–5.

SPR is designed to achieve these goals by facilitating and enhancing core skills through psychoeducation. The intervention evolves through various skill-building steps:

1. Gathering information, identifying current needs, and prioritizing needs and problems to be addressed
2. Building problem-solving skills through focusing on identifying the problem, setting a goal, and choosing the action plan to achieve goals
3. Promoting positive activities through identifying possible constructive activities and scheduling activities
4. Identifying and managing upsetting physical and emotional reactions, and learning new stress- and anxiety-reducing strategies
5. Promoting helpful thinking by extinguishing unhelpful negative thought patterns and promoting helpful, more optimistic patterns of thought
6. Rebuilding healthy social connections by mobilizing family and social supports

For each skill set, alternative methods and approaches are designed to engage children according to their emotional and cognitive levels of development. The provider will link the survivor to the appropriate social and mental health agencies, as needed.

Psychoeducation

Psychoeducation is an intervention used to inform persons about the effects of trauma exposure, bereavement, risk and protective factors, coping strategies, problem-solving skills, and stress management techniques. Psychoeducation may be delivered through a number of venues, which may include one-to-one personal interventions, formal structured presentations, fact sheets delineating expected psychological reactions to disaster, workbooks for children, or electronic media.

The goals of psychoeducation are to normalize disaster reactions, to increase the survivors' sense of control, to help families recognize situations requiring further evaluation or intervention, to encourage children and families to identify and use social supports, and to promote adaptive coping skills (Gard and Ruzek 2006; Young 2006). Psychoeducation can be reassuring for parents by increasing their confidence in their own parenting skills and providing specific guidance on how to support their children (Cohen et al. 2006a). Psychoeducation is an ongoing process throughout all the stages of recovery from trauma exposure.

Parents may need assistance in understanding how to talk with their children about traumatic events. They are encouraged to listen to their children's story of what happened and to respect the children's expression of fears and anxieties. Ideally, parents will be honest in their communications, create a safe environment, empathize with their children, provide reassurance and hopeful expectations, and be supportive and understanding when children briefly regress in their behaviors after exposure to a disaster. Parents should consider sharing their own feelings, encourage children to ask questions, serve as a role model for managing emotions, and maintain household routines around work, eating, sleeping, and recreation.

Parents can help their children identify trustworthy and dependable community helpers, such as police, firefighters, and emergency personnel, and can provide children with emergency numbers and guidance on how to access help. Parents and caretakers are encouraged to minimize children's exposure to traumatic reminders, such as situations, activities, or locations that trigger memories of the disaster. Limits should be placed on television viewing. When children do watch television coverage of the disaster, parents should be present and ready to answer questions. Psychoeducation strategies for children are noted in Table 8–6.

Various Web sites, including those of the American Academy of Child and Adolescent Psychiatry (AACAP; www.aacap.org), the NCTSN (www.nctsnet.org), the American Red Cross (www.redcross.org), and the Federal Emergency Management Agency (FEMA; www.fema.gov), are available as resource centers.

TABLE 8–6. Psychoeducation for parents

- *Gather together as a family.* The best safeguard against disaster stress is the love and support of family members.
- *Reassure the child that he or she is safe.* Let your child know the family will be safe and will stay together.
- *Recognize that children are children.* Younger children may not be able to verbalize their fears and anxieties. When they are afraid, they are most fearful of being left alone. Be sure to include them in your activities before and after an anticipated disaster such as a hurricane.
- *Talk to your child in language that he or she can understand.* Explain to your child what happened, what is happening, and what is going to happen in a language that he or she can understand.
- *Listen to your child's thoughts.* Try to understand how your child thinks and how he or she explains what has happened. Listen and answer questions honestly, but do not volunteer more information than the child needs or is prepared to hear.
- *Listen to your child's feelings.* Listen continuously and reassure a child who is afraid. Try not to minimize or ignore his or her feelings. Where possible, join with your child in understanding his or her feelings, but in a way that conveys that you will manage the situation. Allow your child to mourn or grieve over a lost toy, a missing blanket, and the loss or damage to your home.
- *Encourage your child to talk.* Provide an atmosphere of acceptance in which your child feels free to express his or her anxieties. Include family, friends, or other children in the discussions. Another way of communicating is to have the child draw pictures of the events surrounding the disaster. Have the child tell you about his or her drawings.
- *Routinize and normalize your child's life.* Get back to a routine as quickly as possible. This signifies to your child that you are maintaining control, another sign of adaptive coping. Observing regular meal schedules, planning calming prebedtime activities, and reinstating a bedtime will revitalize family structure and help provide a sense of security for your children.
- *Regulate exposure to disaster imagery.* Limit your child's exposure to the imagery associated with the disaster (television news, newspapers, gratuitous violence, injury, and death). Avoid situations and traumatic reminders that bring back your child's fears.

Psychological Debriefing

Psychological debriefing is a semistructured intervention designed to be carried out after a traumatic event such as a disaster in which survivors are brought together, usually for a single group session, to share their emotional and cognitive understanding of what transpired. The purpose is to promote recovery, normalize reactions, and reconstruct a coherent narrative of the event. A more structured group therapy format known as critical incident stress debriefing provides seven stages through which the traumatic event is discussed from a number of different perspectives, usually within 24–72 hours after the event. No evidence appears in the psychiatric literature, however, to support a policy of a formal, single-session therapeutic intervention for all survivors of a traumatic event, and serious questions have been raised regarding the risk of potential harm for some recipients (Bisson et al. 2007). In some instances, adult survivors may even be retraumatized and have a worsening of their symptoms (Litz and Maguen 2007). Most experts have concluded that little empirical evidence is available to support the use of intensive emotional debriefing in the immediate aftermath of trauma exposure (Orner et al. 2006).

Likewise, limited empirical data are available on psychological debriefing with children, particularly those who have experienced a disaster, and the few pertinent studies have not evaluated the traditional approach to debriefing delivered in a single group session soon after a disaster. Vila et al. (1999) conducted school-based debriefing of children ages 6–9 years 1 day after they had been exposed to a school hostage-taking incident and again 6 weeks later and found that debriefing did not prevent the occurrence of posttraumatic disorders. In a randomized controlled trial of a psychological debriefing format with children ages 7–18 years following road traffic accidents, Stallard et al. (2006) compared a trauma group with a neutral discussion group and failed to find any significant differences, although both groups demonstrated significant gains. Further studies are needed to clarify the conditions under which use of debriefing with children may be facilitative to recovery or harmful for them.

Authors generally agree that group participation should be voluntary, with parental consent; that the survivors should be comparable as to age and degree of exposure (excluding children with traumatic bereavement); and that the intervention should not be employed in the immediate aftermath of disaster when hyperarousal and numbness may be present (Stallard et al. 2006).

Sustained Psychological Interventions

Although most children experiencing posttraumatic stress symptoms will respond to a tincture of time and the various modalities designed to mitigate anxiety, a number of children will have persistent posttraumatic stress symptoms and other coexisting emotional and behavioral problems, such as mood disorder, disruptive behaviors, dissociation, traumatic bereavement, and bodily symptoms, and therefore will require a more sustained treatment program. A number of authors (e.g., Jaycox et al. 2010; Shaw et al. 1996) have noted the persistence of posttraumatic stress symptoms many months after exposure to natural disaster.

Empirical evidence suggests that trauma-informed psychotherapy is efficacious (Silverman et al. 2008). Most empirical studies of psychotherapy have focused on brief CBTs because they have been more readily manualized for research purposes. The mainstream psychosocial approaches are predominantly psychodynamic in nature and usually involve play therapy, family interventions, and group therapies. Although less utilized, CBT has the most empirical evidence to support its use. The choice between individual versus group interventions is determined by the child's clinical presentation, trauma history, and psychological comorbidities, and very frequently by the resources and skilled personnel available.

Cognitive-Behavioral Therapy

Silverman et al. (2008) reviewed 21 psychosocial interventions (1993–2007) for traumatized children and concluded that trauma-focused cognitive-behavioral therapy (TF-CBT) has the most empirical evidence for efficaciousness, followed by school-based group CBT, and the authors concluded that the other interventions were "possibly efficacious." In the "Practice Parameter for the Assessment and Treatment of Children And Adolescents With Posttraumatic Stress Disorder," The AACAP Work Group on Quality Issues identified TF-CBT as the most empirically supported intervention available for use with trauma survivors (Cohen et al. 2010). TF-CBT is a 12- to 16-session intervention designed to be implemented with children ages 4–18 years who have been exposed to any traumatic event. Information regarding this intervention can be obtained from the Center for Traumatic Stress in Children and Adolescents (http://www.wpahs.org/specialties/psychiatry/ctsca).

Cognitive-behavioral interventions are employed in both individual and group formats in various community and school programs (Jaycox et al. 2010), usually over a 10- to 16-week period. CBT approaches include providing information about predictable and expected responses to trauma; engaging children in various exercises to identify and appropriately express emotions; practicing anxiety reduction techniques such as relaxation, focused breathing, positive self-talk, and thought-stopping; discovering the relationship between thoughts, feelings, and behaviors (cognitive restructuring); and guiding children through titrated reexposure using trauma narratives, storytelling, poems, and drawings to help the child slowly achieve mastery over the traumatic situation (Cohen et al. 2006a).

Cognitive processing of the event helps the child to examine and correct misperceptions and distortions. Reconstructing the trauma experience is an integral aspect of processing the event. The goal is to desensitize the child to the trauma event and traumatic reminders so the child can integrate the trauma experience into his or her life (Cohen et al. 2006a). This can be done through talking, in writing, or in the context of art or play. A modification of CBT has been developed for childhood traumatic grief (CBT-CTG; Cohen et al. 2006b), which has been discussed in Chapter 6, "Traumatic Bereavement."

In one study, 24 children, ages 8–18 years, who had experienced a single-incident traumatic event, were randomly assigned to a 10-week CBT intervention or to a waitlist control condition (Smith et al. 2007). At the 6-month follow-up, only one child in the CBT group continued to meet the criteria for posttraumatic stress disorder (PTSD), compared with 60% of the children in the control group, but had experienced improved function and significant reductions in anxiety and depression. In addition to posttraumatic stress symptoms, survivors may develop depressive and other anxiety symptoms related to the cascade of secondary adversities. Other studies have demonstrated the efficacy of behavioral interventions for both anxiety and depression after trauma exposure (Goenjian et al. 1997, 2005). Therapeutic elements in cognitive-behavioral therapies are noted in Table 8–7.

A number of guided activity workbooks designed for children impacted by disaster are available. These include *Helping Children Cope With Disasters* (La Greca et al. 1996), *Healing After Trauma Skills* (Gurwitch and Messenbaugh 2005), and *My Personal Story About Hurricanes Katrina and Rita: A Guided Activity Workbook for Middle and High School Students* (Kliman et al. 2005).

TABLE 8–7. Therapeutic elements in cognitive-behavioral therapies
Psychoeducation
Parenting skills
Anxiety management techniques
Affect modulation
Cognitive restructuring
Exposure therapies
Emotional or information processing therapies
Conjoint child and family sessions
Enhancing safety and future developmental trajectory

Source.   Bisson and Cohen 2006.

Play Therapy

Play has been defined as the child's version of the human ability to deal with experience by creating model situations and mastering reality by experimentation (Erikson 1963). Play is fantasy woven around objects. Play activity has been described as pretend, imaginative, dramatic, spontaneous, self-generated, and an end in itself (Fein 1981). In play, the child's innermost conflicts, concerns, and fears are expressed. Wish fulfillment, expression of pent-up emotions, and experimentation or "trial action" are employed as the child turns passive into active and creates in fantasy what was often absent in reality; these are ways of mastering trauma. Fein (1981) described several childhood activities that meet the criteria of pretend play: 1) familiar activities are performed in the absence of necessary equipment, 2) activities are not carried to their usual outcome, 3) inanimate objects are treated as if they are animate, and 4) the child performs an activity usually performed by an adult.

Play therapy focuses on understanding the meaning that the child places on the trauma experience. Play therapy explores how that experience relates to other childhood experiences, prior traumatic exposures, internal conflicts, defense mechanisms, and coping strategies. Through play, the child may relive and repeat the traumatic situation in fantasy but bring it to a different resolution with a sense of empowerment and mastery (Gillis 1993). After the Chowchilla bus kidnapping, children often played games in which kidnapping occurred and the children in fantasy would triumph over the kidnappers, turning anxiety into mastery

(Terr 1981b). Through play therapy and appropriate interventions, the child learns to deal with the shattering loss of cherished childhood beliefs such as these: "goodness will triumph over evil," "people are inherently good," "parents are powerful and can always protect you," and "I am invulnerable to injury and death" (Shaw 2000).

The therapist interprets the child's thoughts and actions exhibited through play, helping the child to deal with feelings of helplessness experienced during the disaster, integrating the trauma into the child's life experiences, and offering the child new coping strategies (Terr 1981a). Through play activities, children learn to distinguish adaptive and maladaptive coping, enhance resilience, increase self-awareness of internal emotional states, and use empowerment strategies. In some instances, the symbolic repetition of the traumatic situation may result in relief of anxiety as the treatment scenario is mastered, but in other instances, the anxiety may continue unabated (Terr 1981a). The therapist must know when to allow the child to freely express emotions related to the traumatic event and when to clarify meaning, label emotions, and interpret what is being played out. Play therapy has been shown to provide significant clinical improvement for about 75% of children who are treated (Target and Fonagy 1994a, 1994b, 1997).

Guided activity coloring workbooks have been developed for younger children, families, and teachers that allow children to move at their own pace to achieve mastery over traumatic events with adult assistance. Kliman et al. (2001) developed such a manual, *My Book About the Attack on America*, which allows the child to describe memories, perceptions and fears, and to develop positive coping strategies.

Psychopharmacological Interventions

Psychopharmacological interventions are not generally used with children following disaster except for those whose clinical presentation is severe or who have evidence of other simultaneous psychiatric conditions that warrant intervention. The use of psychotropic medications in children should focus on target symptoms, such as agitation, aggressive behaviors, anxiety, and depression, when they impair the child's capacities to meet the ordinary demands of everyday life. Psychopharmacology may be used at any point following disaster.

Psychological reactions to disasters vary from brief psychological distress, which frequently improves without intervention, to more enduring posttraumatic anxiety symptoms that may lead to diagnosed PTSD and other mental disorders.

Adult studies have demonstrated the efficacy of using several classes of medications to treat PTSD. These include selective serotonin reuptake inhibitors (SSRIs), tricyclic antidepressants, α_2-adrenergic agonists, monoamine oxidase inhibitors, second-generation antipsychotics (SGAs), and β-blockers (Baldwin et al. 2005; Foa et al. 2000; Strawn et al. 2010; Van der Kolk 2001). The United Kingdom Committee on Safety of Medicines has suggested that the use of SSRIs is generally acceptable for the treatment of anxiety disorders because the risk of self-harm is minimal and the therapeutic benefits are well documented (Baldwin et al. 2005).

A number of studies have demonstrated the effectiveness of psychotropic medications in the treatment of adult PTSD, but comparable efficaciousness in children and adolescents has not been shown. Although SSRIs are considered to be the first-line drug interventions for adults with PTSD, only limited evidence of their efficaciousness has been found in children and adolescents. In a review of drug interventions for pediatric PTSD, Strawn et al. (2010) identified three double-blind randomized clinical trials (RCTs) of SSRIs, a double-blind RCT of imipramine, and several open-label studies of other medications, such as antiadrenergics, other antidepressants, mood stabilizers, and SGAs. Only one of the three RCTs of SSRIs (sertraline and fluoxetine) suggested a minimal effect, and no differences were noted in the other two studies. A couple of open-trial studies of citalopram in treating pediatric PTSD suggested some efficacy. Although the authors concluded that the data do not support the use of SSRIs as first-line treatment for PTSD in children and adolescents, they suggested that SSRIs have a role with comorbid depressive spectrum disorders and other anxiety disorders.

Other psychopharmacological interventions that have been suggested as possibly having a role in the treatment of pediatric PTSD are antiadrenergic medications (prazosin, clonidine, and guanfacine), β-blockers (propranolol), SGAs (quetiapine and risperidone), and mood stabilizers (carbamazepine and divalproex). Strawn et al. (2010) reported a study that found no differences between propranolol and placebo in preventing PTSD in children (ages 10–18 years) 6 weeks after trauma exposure. Although there have been seven RCTs that demonstrated efficacy of SGAs in the treatment of adult PTSD, there have been only two pediatric PTSD open clinical trials, with risperidone and quetiapine, both of which suggested efficacy. The authors legitimately stressed, however, the risk of significant adverse effects—specifically, extrapyramidal symptoms, hyperlipidemia, and obesity—in patients taking SGAs. Two open-label trials of mood stabilizers (carbamazepine and divalproex) in children and adolescents suggested benefit. Strawn et al. expressed that they are more convinced of the utility of psychopharmacological interventions that directly impact the noradrenergic systems—that is, the antiadrenergics and the SGAs that are potent antagonists at α_1 receptors and that may attenuate posttraumatic stress symptoms and more specifically nightmares and intrusive and hyperarousal symptoms—but further studies are required.

Considerable discussion exists in the adult literature regarding the use of benzodiazepines (Macaluso et al. 2010). Historically, benzodiazepines have been used to manage acute anxiety, mania, agitation, insomnia, and substance withdrawal. However, debate continues regarding their use in anxiety disorders. Adverse effects associated with their use include sedation, fatigue, ataxia, forgetfulness, and disinhibition. In treating PTSD, benzodiazepines are generally recognized to reduce distress and promote sleep but not to improve the core symptoms, such as nightmares, or to affect the course of the illness (Van der Kolk 2001). Other adult studies have suggested that use of benzodiazepines may even increase the risk of PTSD (Gelpin et al. 1996)

Donnelly et al. (1999) suggested that children with PTSD are more likely to manifest additional psychiatric conditions such as depression (Giaconia et al. 1995; Sack et al. 1995), anxiety disorders (Giaconia et al. 1995; Kinzie et al. 1986), and disruptive behaviors, including attention-deficit/hyperactivity disorder, conduct disorder, substance abuse, and oppositional defiant disorder (McLeer et al. 1998; Steiner et al. 1997). It is often the presence of coexisting psychiatric disorders that leads to psychopharmacological intervention.

Family Interventions

The traumatized child should, whenever possible, be treated in conjunction with family members. In that sense, all interventions with children are ideally family interventions. The effect of the traumatic stressor on the family influences the child's psychological response, and the child's response simultaneously impacts the family's adaptation to trauma. The family's reaction to a traumatic event is shaped by the nature of the stressors and the reactions of individual family members and is mediated by the family's religious, ethnic, and cultural beliefs. As a caretaking unit for the child, the family is challenged by the experience of traumatic exposure, death, and separation from loved ones. Family and parental support can mitigate the child's risk for developing posttraumatic stress symptoms. Conversely, the presence of poor family functioning or of parents with psychological disorders predicts elevated levels of psychological disorders in the children (AACAP 1998).

The efficacy of family interventions following trauma exposure remains to be proved (Miller 2003). Several studies that have attempted to supplement child-focused CBT for anxiety disorders with family CBT have not convincingly demonstrated incremental efficacy for the family component (Barrett et al. 1996; Cobham et al. 1998; Spence et al. 2000). However, Wood et al. (2006) compared child-focused CBT with family-focused CBT (12–16 sessions) for children, ages 6–13 years, with anxiety disorders (no PTSD) and found that compared with the child approach, the family approach was associated with decreased severity of the anxiety disorder coupled with improved social and school functioning.

Berkowitz et al. (2010b) developed the Child and Family Traumatic Stress Intervention (CFTSI), a brief therapy designed for families with children ages 7–17 that is implemented in the wake of trauma exposure. Four sessions of CFTSI are delivered in the family home or in an office setting. CFTSI involves extensive reporting on symptoms and feelings. CFTSI is intended to decrease the negative impact of children's exposure to traumatic events and serves concurrently as an assessment and engagement strategy as well as a secondary prevention intervention. The goals of CFTSI are to prevent a child from developing posttraumatic symptoms and to increase the likelihood that children will actively engage in and sustain participation in longer-term treatments when these are indicated. CFTSI seeks to enhance family communication and support for the trauma-exposed child through the following approaches:

- Increasing the level of understanding of the impact of trauma exposure on symptoms, behavior changes, and daily functioning
- Increasing the child's ability to communicate feelings and symptoms to the parent
- Increasing parents' ability to respond appropriately and supportively to the child's difficulties by teaching parents strategies to use with their child
- Providing case management and care coordination related to trauma exposure
- Helping the family access needed services and maintain parents' focus on their children rather than on the external stressors associated with the traumatic event

In a comparison study with a supportive group intervention, CFTSI was superior in reducing posttraumatic stress symptoms (Berkowitz et al. 2010b).

Treating Youth With Substance Abuse and Traumatic Stress

Traumatized adolescents who have turned to substance abuse to miti-gate the psychological effects of trauma represent a challenge to mental health professionals because their clinical presentation is characterized by more severe and diverse maladaptive behaviors. Table 8–8 lists ap-proaches proposed by NCTSN (2008) for treating adolescents with sus-pected substance abuse.

TABLE 8–8. Therapeutic approaches for youth with posttraumatic stress disorder and substance abuse

---

Include assessments of substance abuse problems and traumatic stress as part of routine screening/assessment procedures.

Establish a therapeutic relationship that is consistent, trusting, and collaborative.

Provide psychoeducation for both youth and their families about trauma and substance abuse problems.

Encourage parental involvement in treatment with the goal of increasing parenting skills, communication, and conflict resolution.

Emphasize management and reduction of both substance use and posttraumatic stress disorder symptoms early in the recovery process.

Initiate relapse prevention efforts early, targeting both substance and trauma-related cues (e.g., problem-solving, drug refusal, and safety skills; desensitization to trauma reminders).

Emphasize stress management skills, such as relaxation and positive self-talk.

Teach cognitive restructuring techniques, such as recognizing, challenging, and correcting negative cognitions.

Provide social skills training.

Consider whether treatment requires random urine drug screens to monitor abstinence.

Consider referral to adolescent self-help groups as needed.

Employ, when indicated, adjunct psychopharmacological treatment to relieve acute symptoms of drug withdrawal or traumatic stress.

Make use of school-based treatment programs to reach at-risk youth.

Source.   National Child Traumatic Stress Network 2008.

Seeking Safety, an integrated treatment approach for co-occurring substance abuse disorder and PTSD in adults, has been developed by Najavits, who noted that having both active substance abuse and PTSD creates an urgent need to establish safety (Najavits 2002). The intent of the approach is to reduce self-harm behaviors, dangerous relationships, risky behaviors, and drug-using friends, and to gain self-control over self-destructive behaviors. The intervention has 25 modules, divided among cognitive, behavioral, and interpersonal themes, that can be used in the treatment program. Applying Seeking Safety to an adolescent population requires sensitivity to cognitive and emotional development and to issues of confidentiality and self-disclosure, and may require limited parental involvement (with the adolescent's permission). When implemented with adolescents, Seeking Safety has demonstrated greater improvements than has treatment as usual in substance abuse domains, PTSD cognitions, and levels of deviant behavior.

Community Interventions

Systems of Care

Community-based interventions following disaster involve setting up a system of care for the benefit of children and their families (Cohen et al. 2010). *System of care* refers to a comprehensive network of mental health services, child-serving programs, and natural community support services organized to meet the needs of children and families. Ursano and Friedman (2006) have suggested that disaster mental health care requires a systematic approach that integrates a community-level public health focus with an individualized clinical treatment focus. Systems of care represent an organized effort to integrate government-, community-, and school-based services that are sensitive to the needs of the family, individualized to meet the child's needs, and delivered in the least restrictive environment.

Community resilience is a measure of the rapidity and efficacy with which a community recovers from disaster. For a community to be resilient, its members must work together to quickly take effective actions to respond to emerging adversities. The best contributions to the resilience of a community involve preparation for and anticipation of the consequences of disaster. If residents, agencies, and organizations take meaningful and intentional actions before an event, they can help the community reestablish stability after the event. Resilience implies that after an event, a community not only may be able to cope and to recover, but also may change to reflect different priorities arising from the disaster. To be most effective, community plans must address the emotional well-being of residents, families, and their children. The NCTSN has put together a guidebook that provides information about building community resilience aimed at helping communities improve their capacity to respond effectively to natural or human-made disasters or acts of terrorism (Gurwitch et al. 2007).

Social Support

Social support has been defined as the "social interactions that provide individuals with actual assistance and embed them into a web of social relationships perceived to be loving, caring and readily available in times of need" (Kaniasty 2005, p. 1). The presence of strong and available social support has been documented to mitigate both acute and long-term mental health effects of trauma (Kaniasty 2005; Pine and Cohen 2002). Children's development is influenced, beyond the family sphere, by continuous interaction with peers, teachers, community members, and mass media. Through social interactions, children internalize culturally constructed norms, values, and beliefs, including acceptable social behaviors and modes of expressing emotion. Children's development is inextricably connected to surrounding social and cultural influences, particularly the families and communities that function as the children's life-support systems.

Using available social supports is a helpful strategy in a community-based shelter or disaster recovery setting. If individuals are disconnected from their usual sources of social support, they should be encouraged to make use of immediately available options (disaster responders, health care professionals, relief workers, other survivors in the shelter environment), while remaining respectful of individual preferences (NCTSN and NCPTSD 2006).

School-Based Interventions

School-age children are more likely than adults to manifest impairment after disaster (Wolmer et al. 2005). One of the most effective and expeditious interventions for child survivors of disaster is *rapid restoration of an operating school system*. Teachers are well versed in working with children, often during periods of crisis, and are trusted by students and parents as caretakers. They know the children and are thus well able to assess significant changes in the child's behavior.

A school-based behavioral health response plan should include assessment strategies to identify children at risk and to distinguish whether these children can be managed in the school setting or require referral to community mental health professionals. Subsequent to disaster, intervention teams composed of mental health professionals and crisis intervention specialists are formed and assigned to specific schools or regions to assist the school in assessment and intervention programs. In the school community, it is essential to address the emotional needs of teachers, counselors, and school administrators who not only interact daily with the disaster-affected children and their families, but also are themselves survivors of the same disaster.

The school system is often staffed with counselors and crisis intervention specialists who are able to identify children at risk and intervene when necessary on behalf of children and their families. For example, 58% of children seen for counseling after the 9/11 attacks were managed in the school setting (Stuber et al. 2002). Schools can implement programs and create opportunities for children to connect with each other and share their experiences. In addition, schools provide routine academic tasks requiring focused attention, as well as opportunities for success experiences that help facilitate resilience and recovery. Following a disaster, schools disseminate accurate disaster recovery information, provide health care for students, and distribute life-sustaining supplies.

School-based interventions following disaster provide opportunities to normalize psychological reactions, clarify what happened, correct cognitive distortions, facilitate children's expressing of fears and worries, encourage peer interactions, and identify children in need of further assessment and referral. School-based interventions can also reduce psychological morbidity after disaster. A teacher-based, resilience-focused, stress-inoculation training program, administered to fourth and fifth graders who were later exposed to 3 weeks of continuing rocket and mortar attacks in Israel, was found to lead to significantly lower symptoms of PTSD and stress/mood symptoms in the intervention group than in the control group (Wolmer et al. 2011).

A manualized treatment intervention, Cognitive Behavioral Intervention for Trauma in Schools (CBITS; Jaycox 2004), has been developed for the school setting. This group intervention for children, usually in grades 5–9, is designed to mitigate children's posttraumatic stress symptoms, depression, and anxiety through teaching of positive coping skills, relaxation techniques, cognitive reframing, and social problem solving, and through homework assignments. A study comparing CBITS in a school setting with TF-CBT in a mental health clinic found the treatments equally efficacious, but children were more likely to accept treatment offered in the school setting (98%) than in the mental health clinic (37%) (Jaycox et al. 2010).

The RAND Corporation has developed the tool kit *How Schools Can Help Students Recover From Traumatic Experiences: A Tool Kit for Supporting Long-Term Recovery* (Jaycox et al. 2006). This publication helps schools choose a trauma recovery program that best fits the students' needs.

The Federal Response

The federal government is responsible for a number of initiatives and programs designed to provide relief to the survivors of disaster. The Disaster Relief Act of 1974 established FEMA to have responsibility for coordinating the federal response. In 2003, FEMA became a part of the newly formed Department of Homeland Security (DHS). Federal involvement occurs after a major disaster has overwhelmed local resources and the state requests such assistance. Once the President declares a major disaster, a federal-state agreement is prepared to delineate the types of assistance to be provided and the areas eligible for assistance. Programs are initiated to provide support for individuals experiencing mild to moderate psychological stress and to facilitate recovery. A principal federal official is appointed by DHS to oversee the disaster response, including local, state, and federal governmental disaster resources, and the coordination of voluntary disaster relief agencies, such as the Red Cross and Salvation Army.

Disaster mental health services are provided through the Emergency Services and Disaster Relief Branch of the Center for Mental Health Services (CMHS) within the Substance Abuse and Mental Health Services Administration (SAMHSA). The Stafford Act provides funding for training and services to implement psychological services. Grants are provided by FEMA through two CMHS programs: 1) the Immediate Services Program, which provides funds for screening, diagnostic, and counseling outreach services for up to 60 days, and 2) the Regular Services Program, which funds crisis counseling, community outreach, and consultation to assist people affected by disaster. The network of public and private community mental health centers and academic institutions provides education and training to crisis intervention specialists, who are mobilized at times of disaster.

The American Red Cross, an independent humanitarian organization, is privately funded and mandated by Congress to have a central and unique role in disaster response. The organization provides designated mass care venues for disaster survivors to obtain psychosocial interventions and psychoeducation.

When acts of terrorism occur, the Federal Bureau of Investigation has the primary responsibility for spearheading the crisis management of the event. "Consequence management" includes measures to protect public health and safety, restore essential government services, and provide emergency relief to government, businesses, and individuals affected by the terrorist act (Siegrist and Graham 1999). The Department of Health and Human Services (HHS) assumes major responsibility for the medical, public health, and mental health emergency support activities, including coordination with state and local governments in providing resources to the community.

The National Commission on Children and Disasters (2010) presented a number of recommendations focused on the mental health of children:

1. HHS should take the lead to integrate children's mental and behavioral health into public health, medical, and other relevant disaster management activities.
2. HHS should enhance research endeavors focused on the efficacy of intervention strategies and programs to enhance children's resilience following disasters.
3. Federal agencies and nonfederal partners should enhance predisaster preparedness and enhance training in Psychological First Aid, bereavement support, and brief supportive interventions.
4. DHS/FEMA and SAMHSA should strengthen the government's Crisis Counseling Assistance and Training Program.
5. Congress should establish a single, flexible grant-funding mechanism to support the delivery of mental health treatment services that address the full spectrum of children's behavioral health needs.

■ Key Clinical Points

- ■ Evidence-based science has begun to identify the most promising interventions for use with disaster survivors.

- ■ Interventions are provided in a staged sequence across a timeline.

- ■ Community-based systems involving school, social supports, and nonfederal and federal agencies are critical in responding to the needs of individuals and their families.

- ■ Psychological debriefing should be used with caution.

- ■ Psychological First Aid is administered in the immediate aftermath of disaster.

- ■ Skills for Psychological Recovery is an intervention administered in the intermediate aftermath of disaster.

- ■ Crisis intervention strategies, psychoeducation, and other focused stress-reduction interventions may be used for persons with continuing distress.

- ■ More sustained manualized interventions, such as cognitive-behavioral therapy, are employed for more defined emotional and behavioral disorders such as PTSD.

- ■ School-based interventions have an important role in postdisaster interventions.

- ■ Medications may be prescribed on an individual basis according to specific clinical indications.

References

American Academy of Child and Adolescent Psychiatry: Practice parameter for the assessment and treatment of children and adolescents with posttraumatic stress disorder. J Am Acad Child Adolesc Psychiatry 37:4S–26S, 1998

Auerbach SM, Kilmann PR: Crisis intervention: a review of outcomes research. Psychol Bull 84:1189–1217, 1977

Baldwin DS, Anderson IM, Nutt DJ, et al: Evidence-based guidelines for the pharmacological treatment of anxiety disorders: recommendations from the British Association of Psychopharmacology. J Psychopharmacol 19:567–596, 2005

Barrett PM, Dadds MR, Rapee RM: Family treatment of childhood anxiety: a controlled study. J Consult Clin Psychol 64:333–342, 1996

Berkowitz S, Bryant R, Brymer M, et al; National Center for PTSD and the National Child Traumatic Stress Network: Skills for Psychological Recovery: Field Operations Guide. Washington, DC, National Center for PTSD and National Child Traumatic Stress Network, 2010a

Berkowitz S, Stover CS, Marans SR: The Child and Family Traumatic Stress Intervention: secondary prevention for youth at risk of developing PTSD. J Child Psychol Psychiatry 52:676–685, 2010b

Bisson JI, Cohen JA: Disseminating early interventions following trauma. J Trauma Stress 19:583–595, 2006

Bisson JI, Brayne M, Ochberg FM, et al: Early psychosocial intervention following traumatic events. Am J Psychiatry 164:1016–1019, 2007

Cobham VE, Dadds MR, Spence SH: The role of parental anxiety in the treatment of childhood anxiety. J Consult Clin Psychol 66:893–905, 1998

Cohen JA, Mannarino AP, Gibson LE, et al: Interventions for children and adolescents following disaster, in Interventions Following Mass Violence and Disasters. Edited by Ritchie EC, Watson PJ, Friedman MJ. New York, Guilford, 2006a, pp 227–256

Cohen JA, Mannarino AP, Staron VR: A pilot study of modified cognitive behavioral therapy for childhood traumatic grief. J Am Acad Child Adolesc Psychiatry 45:1465–1473, 2006b

Cohen JA, Bukstein O, Walter H, et al; American Academy of Child and Adolescent Psychiatry Work Group on Quality Issues: Practice parameter for the assessment and treatment of children and adolescents with posttraumatic stress disorder. J Am Acad Child Adolesc Psychiatry 49:414–430, 2010

Donnelly CL, Amaya-Jackson L, March J: Psychopharmacology of pediatric posttraumatic stress disorder. J Am Acad Child Adolesc Psychiatry 9:203–220, 1999

Erikson E: Childhood and Society, 2nd Edition. New York, Norton, 1963

Fein GF: Pretend play in childhood: an integrative review. Child Dev 52:1095–1118, 1981

Foa EB, Keane TM, Friedman MJ: Guidelines for treatment of PTSD. J Trauma Stress 13:539–588, 2000

Gard BA, Ruzek JI: Community mental health response to crisis. J Clin Psychol 62:1029–1041, 2006

Gelpin E, Bonne O, Peri T, et al: Treatment of recent trauma survivors with benzodiazepines: a prospective study. J Clin Psychiatry 57:390–394, 1996

Giaconia RM, Reinherz HZ, Silverman AB, et al: Traumas and posttraumatic stress disorder in a community population of older adolescents. J Am Acad Child Adolesc Psychiatry 34:1369–1380, 1995

Gillis HM: Individual and small group psychotherapy for children involved in trauma and disaster, in Children and Disaster. Edited by Saylor CF. New York, Plenum, 1993, pp 165–186

Goenjian AK, Karayan I, Pynoos RS, et al: Outcome of psychotherapy among early adolescents after trauma. Am J Psychiatry 154:536–542, 1997

Goenjian AK, Walling D, Steinberg AM, et al: A prospective study of posttraumatic stress and depressive reactions among treated and untreated adolescents 5 years after a catastrophic disaster. Am J Psychiatry 162:2302–2308, 2005

Gurwitch RH, Messenbaugh AK: Healing After Trauma Skills: A Manual for Professionals, Teachers, and Families Working With Children After Trauma/ Disaster, 2nd Edition. 2005. Available at: www.nctsnet.org/nctsn_assets/pdfs/edu_materials/HATS2ndEdition.pdf. Accessed January 20, 2010.

Gurwitch RH, Pfefferbaum B, Montgomery JM, et al: Building Community Resilience for Children and Families. Oklahoma City, Terrorism and Disaster Center at the University of Oklahoma Health Sciences Center, 2007

Jaycox L: Cognitive-Behavioral Intervention for Trauma in Schools. Longmont, CO, Sopris West, 2004

Jaycox LH, Morse LK, Tanielian T, et al: How Schools Can Help Students Recover From Traumatic Experiences: A Tool Kit for Supporting Long-Term Recovery. Santa Monica, CA, RAND Corporation, 2006

Jaycox LH, Cohen JA, Manarino AP, et al: Children's mental health care following Hurricane Katrina: a field trial of trauma-focused psychotherapies. J Trauma Stress 23:223–231, 2010

Kaniasty K: Social support and traumatic stress. PTSD Research Quarterly 16:1–7, 2005

Kinzie JD, Sack WH, Angell RH, et al: The psychiatric effects of massive trauma on Cambodian children. J Am Acad Child Adolesc Psychiatry 25:370–376, 1986

Kliman G, Oklan E, Wolfe H: My Book About the Attack on America. San Francisco, CA, Children's Psychological Trauma Center, 2001

Kliman G, Oklan, E, Wolfe, H, et al: My Personal Story About Hurricanes Katrina and Rita: A Guided Activity Workbook for Middle and High School Students. San Francisco, Children's Psychological Health Center, 2005

Koss MP, Butcher JN: Research on brief psychotherapy, in Handbook of Psychotherapy and Behavior. Edited by Garfield SL, Bergin AE. New York, Wiley, 1986, pp 627–670

La Greca AM, Vernberg EM, Silverman WK, et al: Helping Children Cope With Disasters: A Manual for Professionals Working With Elementary School Children. Miami, University of Miami and Florida International University, 1996

Lindemann E: Symptomatology and management of acute grief. Am J Psychiatry 101:141–148, 1944

Litz BT, Maguen S: Early intervention for trauma, in Handbook of PTSD: Science and Practice. Edited by Friedman MJ, Keane TM, Resnick PA. New York, Guilford, 2007, pp 306–329

Macaluso, M, Kalia R, Faryal S, et al: The role of benzodiazepines in the treatment of anxiety disorders: a clinical review. Psychiatr Ann 40:605–610, 2010

McLeer SV, Dixon JF, Henry D, et al: Psychopathology in non-clinically referred sexually abused children. J Am Acad Child Adolesc Psychiatry 37:1326–1333, 1998

Miller L: Family therapy of terroristic trauma: psychological syndromes and treatment strategies. Am J Fam Ther 31:257–280, 2003

Mitchell JT: When disaster strikes: the critical incident stress debriefing process. JEMS 8:36–39, 1983

Najavits LM: Seeking Safety: A Treatment Manual for PTSD and Substance Abuse. New York, Guilford, 2002

National Child Traumatic Stress Network: Understanding the Links Between Adolescent Trauma and Substance Abuse: A Toolkit for Providers, 2nd Edition. June 2008. Available at: www.nctsn.org/sites/default/files/assets/pdfs/satoolkit_providerguide.pdf. Accessed September 3, 2011.

National Child Traumatic Stress Network and National Center for PTSD: Psychological First Aid Field Operations Guide, 2nd Edition. 2006. Available at: www.nctsn.org/content/psychological-first-aid. Accessed August 16, 2011.

National Commission on Children and Disasters: 2010 Report to the President and Congress (AHRQ Publ No 10-M037). Rockville, MD, Agency for Healthcare Research and Quality, October 2010

National Institute of Mental Health: Mental health and mass violence: Evidence-based early psychological intervention for victims/survivors of mass violence. A workshop to reach consensus on best practices (NIH Publ No 02-5138). Washington, DC, U.S. Government Printing Office, 2002

Orner RJ, Kent AT, Pfefferbaum B, et al: The context of providing immediate postevent intervention, in Interventions Following Mass Violence and Disasters. Edited by Ritchie EC, Watson PJ, Friedman MJ. New York, Guilford Press, 2006, pp 121–133

Pine OS, Cohen JA: Trauma in children and adolescents: risk and treatment of psychiatric sequelae. Biol Psychiatry 51:519–531, 2002

Pynoos RS, Nader K: Psychological first aid and treatment approach to children exposed to community violence. J Trauma Stress 1:445–473, 1988

Reissman DB, Watson PJ, Klomp RW, et al: Prior SD: Pandemic influenza preparedness: adaptive responses to an evolving challenge. Journal of Homeland Security and Emergency Management 3(2), article 13, 2006

Sack W, Clarks G, Seeley J: Posttraumatic stress disorder across two generations of Cambodian refugees. J Am Acad Child Adolesc Psychiatry 34:1160–1166, 1995

Shaw JA: Children, adolescents and trauma. Psychiatr Q 71:227–243, 2000

Shaw JA, Applegate B, Schorr C: Twenty-one-month follow-up study of school-age children exposed to Hurricane Andrew. J Am Acad Child Adolesc Psychiatry 35:359–364, 1996

Siegrist DW, Graham JM (eds): Countering Biological Terrorism in the U.S.: An Understanding of Issues and Status. Dobbs Ferry, NY, Oceana Publications, 1999

Silverman WK, Ortiz CD, Viswesvaran C, et al. Evidence-based psychosocial treatments for children and adolescents exposed to traumatic events. J Clin Child Adolesc Psychol 37:156–183, 2008

Smith P, Yule W, Perrin S, et al: Cognitive-behavioral therapy for PTSD in children and adolescents: a preliminary randomized controlled trial. J Am Acad Child Adolesc Psychiatry 46:1051–1061, 2007

Spence SH, Donovan C, Brechman-Toussaint M: The treatment of childhood social phobia: the effectiveness of a social skills training-based, cognitive-behavioural intervention, with and without parental involvement. J Child Psychol Psychiatry 41:713–726, 2000

Stallard P, Velleman R, Salter E, et al: A randomized controlled trial to determine the effectiveness of an early psychological intervention with children involved in road traffic accidents. J Child Psychol Psychiatry 47:127–134, 2006

Steiner H, Garcia IG, Matthews Z: Posttraumatic stress disorder in incarcerated juvenile delinquents. J Am Acad Child Adolesc Psychiatry 36:357–365, 1997

Strawn JR, Keeshin BR, DelBello MP, et al: Psychopharmacologic treatment of posttraumatic stress disorder in children and adolescents: a review. J Clin Psychiatry 71:932–941, 2010

Stuber J, Fairbrother G, Galea S, et al: Determinants of counseling for children in Manhattan after the September 11 attacks. Psychiatr Serv 53:815–822, 2002

Target M, Fonagy P: Efficacy of psychoanalysis for children with emotional disorders. J Am Acad Child Adolesc Psychiatry 33:361–367, 1994a

Target M, Fonagy P: The efficacy of psychoanalysis for children: prediction of outcome in a developmental context. J Am Acad Child Adolesc Psychiatry 33:1134–1144, 1994b

Target M, Fonagy P: Research on intensive psychotherapy with children and adolescents. Child Adolesc Psychiatr Clin N Am 6:39–51, 1997

Terr LC: Forbidden games, posttraumatic child's play. J Am Acad Child Adolesc Psychiatry 20:741–760, 1981a

Terr L: Psychic trauma in children: observations following the Chowchilla school bus kidnappings. Am J Psychiatry 138:14–19, 1981b

Ursano R, Friedman MJ: Mental health and behavioral interventions for victims of disasters and mass violence, in Interventions Following Mass Violence and Disasters. Edited by Ritchie EC, Watson PJ, Friedman MJ. New York, Guilford, 2006, pp 405–414

Van der Kolk BA: The psychology and psychopharmacology of PTSD. Hum Psychopharmacol 16 (suppl 1):S49–S64, 2001

Vila G, Porche LM, Mouren-Simeoni MC: An 18-month longitudinal study of posttraumatic disorders in children who were taken hostage in their school. Psychosom Med 61:746–754, 1999

Wolmer L, Laor N, Dedeoglu C, et al: Teacher-mediated intervention after disaster: a controlled three-year follow-up of children's functioning. J Child Psychol Psychiatry 46:1161–1168, 2005

Wolmer L, Hamiel D, Laor N: Preventing children's posttraumatic stress after disaster with teacher-based intervention: a controlled study. J Am Acad Child Adolesc Psychiatry 50:340–348, 2011

Wood JJ, Piacentini JC, Southam-Gerow M, et al: Family cognitive behavioral therapy for child anxiety disorders. J Am Acad Child Adolesc Psychiatry 45:314–321, 2006

Young BH: The immediate response to disaster: guidelines for adult psychological first aid, in Interventions Following Mass Violence and Disasters. Edited by Ritchie EC, Watson PJ, Friedman MJ. New York, Guilford, 2006, pp 134–154

9

Generally Accepted Truths

The Psychological Effects of Trauma on Children

Each disaster event produces a defining *trauma signature* with its unique constellation of risk factors. Each disaster event produces a novel array of stressors and risk factors for psychological morbidity both during the impact phase and in its aftermath.

Children's emotional and behavioral responses to stressful situations are often less intense than might be anticipated. Children and adolescents manifest considerable resilience in the face of trauma. The degree and dose of trauma exposure are the major determinants of psychological morbidity. A complex array of mediators shape and determine resilience in children and adolescents.

Children's psychological responses to trauma vary with age and cognitive development. Preschool children usually manifest sleep and appetite disturbance, clinging dependence, and regressive behaviors. School-age children commonly exhibit specific fears, separation anxiety, sleep and behavior problems, play reenactments, somatic complaints, decrements in academic performance, and the more classical spectrum of posttraumatic stress symptoms. In addition to having posttraumatic stress symptoms, adolescents are more likely to be concerned with the life unlived, have dependence-independence conflicts, experience identity issues, and be at risk for misuse of substances.

Certain psychological responses to trauma occur regardless of the nature of the trauma exposure. Regardless of the nature of a disaster and the varied threats of bodily injury and death, victims experience a similar core of posttraumatic stress symptoms, including emotional distress, fears of recurrence, alterations to interpersonal and social life, and a paradoxical proclivity to reexperience and to avoid images, cognitions, and affects associated with the trauma, often with symptoms of hyperarousal.

Exposure to a traumatic stressor may occur through direct and immediate physical impact, on-scene witnessing of the event, media exposure, or interpersonal connectedness to disaster victims. Proximity and dose have a differential effect on the degree of psychological morbidity.

Combined forms of exposure increase risk for psychological consequences. Children exposed to multiple adversities have an increased risk of posttraumatic stress symptoms and poorer psychosocial adjustment and adaptation.

Previous trauma exposure increases vulnerability to subsequent trauma exposure. Repeated trauma exposure, even across different categories of trauma, increases the likelihood of posttraumatic stress symptomatology. For example, children exposed to a tsunami, war-related trauma, and family violence are more likely to suffer from the cumulative effect of trauma exposure and, as a consequence, experience more problems with psychosocial adjustment and adaptation than are children exposed to one of the trauma types.

Repetitive exposure to a *distant* trauma through television and media viewing increases risks for posttraumatic stress symptoms. Children who view media images of distant events, such as the *Challenger* explosion, the 9/11 terrorist attacks, and the Oklahoma City bombing, may exhibit posttraumatic stress symptomatology secondary to media exposure.

Compared with exposure to natural disasters or nonintentional human-generated traumatic events, exposure to intentional human-generated trauma and disaster is associated with greater risk for psychological impairment and illness. Children exposed to interpersonal or mass violence against others experience higher rates of and more severe psychological morbidity.

War is characterized by chronic and enduring exposure to trauma-related events for children and families. The greater the dose and intensity of war-related trauma exposure, the greater is the likelihood of psychological morbidity and problems with psychosocial adjustment and poorer adaptation.

A disaster or extreme event may set in motion a cascade of secondary stressors and effectively transform an acute traumatic situation into an

enduring process of responding to secondary adversities. Although the impact phase of a disaster may be brief (hours to days) and is often circumscribed in time and space, the aftermath of disaster may result in a succession of secondary stressors, such as shortages of basic necessities, devastated community infrastructure, displacement from home and shelter, loss of valued possessions, school closures, disruption of health care services, unemployment, and economic crisis.

The term *complex trauma* refers to repeated trauma exposure that begins in childhood and accumulates throughout the developmental years. The consequences of complex trauma exposure may include difficulties with emotional instability, problems with social and interpersonal relations, mood dysregulation, altered systems of meanings, negative self-attributions, and diminished self-efficacy. The psychological effects of the trauma experiences are woven into the very fabric of personality structure and increase the child's vulnerability to future trauma.

Trauma impacts not only the individual child but also the family and social system within which the child lives. The effect of the traumatic stressor on the family influences the child's psychological response. Reciprocally, the child's response impacts the family's adaptation to trauma. The family reaction to a traumatic event is shaped by the nature of the stressors and the reactions of individual family members and is mediated by the family's religious, ethnic, and cultural beliefs.

The parents' level of function and their symptoms predict the expression of posttraumatic stress symptoms in children. The child's emotional and behavioral responses, including posttraumatic stress symptoms, often mirror those of the parents.

The child's subjective experience of a traumatic situation at the time of exposure is a powerful predictor of the child's psychological outcome. How one defines a situation determines one's emotional response. Child survivors who experience panic, dissociation, or overwhelming feelings of hopelessness are at greater risk for subsequent psychological morbidity.

The risk of posttraumatic stress symptoms increases for both children and adults who are physically injured or who have a family member injured or killed. Children who are injured while exposed to war-related trauma or a national disaster are more likely to experience posttraumatic stress symptoms than are uninjured children.

The psychological response to a traumatic situation may be delayed (sleeper effect) and may worsen over time. The sleeper effect has also been noted in children exposed to disaster, but the effect is difficult to separate from ongoing exposure to secondary adversities.

Traumatic reminders are internal and external triggers that suddenly bring the traumatic event back into awareness with all its emotional, perceptual, and ideational content. Exposure to traumatic reminders results in a resurfacing of posttraumatic stress symptoms. Usually, a gradual habituation effect occurs, with decreasing psychological distress over time.

The psychological effects of earlier trauma exposure in childhood add to a child's psychological or psychiatric vulnerability to disaster. Early exposure to family or community violence, parental death, child maltreatment, or life-impairing or life-threatening medical illness increases the child's risk for posttraumatic stress symptoms and other psychological morbidities with subsequent trauma exposure.

The existence of community solidarity and social cohesion before and after disaster favorably affects the course of posttraumatic stress. Communities with a strong sense of cohesion and shared values suffer less psychiatric morbidity compared with communities lacking such solidarity.

Careful assessment of children's psychological reactions is essential for identifying children at elevated risk for disaster-related psychosocial consequences and children with a diagnosable mental disorder in need of therapeutic interventions. In addition to having posttraumatic stress symptoms, children may experience a spectrum of internalizing, externalizing, and somatic symptoms/mental disorders associated with the losses and secondary adversities that occur in the aftermath of disaster.

Because disasters impact the child while living in a family and a community, interventions are tailored for application not only to the child but also to the family and the encompassing community. Contagion of emotionality and reciprocity of emotional affects occur between members of a family or social group.

Cognitive-behavioral intervention techniques have the greatest empirical evidence regarding efficacy for treating posttraumatic stress symptoms for persons exposed to trauma and disaster. Trauma-focused cognitive behavioral therapy (TF-CBT) and cognitive-behavioral interventions have been found to be efficacious for use with trauma survivors.

Index

Page numbers printed in **boldface** *type refer to tables or figures.*